Praise for *Drink L*

"*Drink Less; Live Better* is a definitive guide to mind, body and soul recovery, set out in a readable and relatable collection of stories, insights and teachings that inspire thought, action and transformation."

William Porter – Author of *Alcohol Explained*

"Get this book, it might just save your life. Sarah is not only a fantastic coach and podcaster, she is now an incredible author. LOVE THIS BOOK! Sarah has a way with words that shines through her podcast and now onto the page. Sarah is now the queen of quit-lit, a must-read! Fabulous!"

Andy Ramage – Author of
The 28 Day Alcohol Free Challenge and *Let's Do This*

"Sarah is not only an incredible human being, but she's also a highly skilled and empathetic coach. Her book *Drink Less; Live Better* is a testament to her expertise and passion for helping people improve their lives. Through her insightful and practical approach, Sarah shares valuable strategies that worked for her on her journey to drink less and live a more fulfilling life, then provides actions for the readers at the end of each chapter. Her powerful insights will help countless people learn more about themselves and create positive change in their lives. We highly recommend this book to anyone seeking to improve their relationship with alcohol and live a happier, healthier life. Thank you, Sarah, for sharing your wisdom and expertise with the world!"

Alex Walker and Lisa Elsworth – Founders of Bee Sober

"Each turn of the page brings forth a fresh wave of inspiration, reminding us all of the immeasurable strength we have. Within these chapters, you will discover a treasure trove – an invitation to embrace the limitless possibilities of recovery and to find solace in the stories of someone else. May this book ignite a spark within you, guiding you towards your own pathway of joyous recovery and reminding you that, even in the face of adversity, joy can prevail."

Naetha Uren RCPF – CEO Recovery Coach Academy

"This book is a fabulous resource for those who wish to address their relationship with alcohol. It draws on Sarah's own experiences as well as her work as a certified sober coach.

Her non-patronising approach makes this book relatable, and very easy to dip in and out of as you negotiate your own path to either moderation or sobriety.

Let Sarah guide, support and nourish you as you start to put yourself first and give yourself the future you deserve."

Lea Watson – Glow Sober

"Sarah has enormous capacity of humour, heart and wisdom and I am delighted and lucky to count her among my most treasured friends as well as most respected colleagues. She is a bright (incredibly so, wear your sunglasses) light in the worlds of sobriety, well-being and life lived out loud."

Jo Anne Walduck – Recovery, business and life coach

"Farewell to autopilot drinking (and all the low vibes that go with it)! Sarah is a sweet angel on your shoulder, gently and firmly reminding you that you don't need that drink to de-stress/unwind/have a good time."

Kelly Pietangeli – www.myprojectme.com

"Not only has Sarah been an amazing friend, supporting me and walking side by side with me along the sober journey, she's also been an incredible leader within my community. Sarah's led insightful workshops, written inspiring columns and offered incredible assistance to so many. I have no doubt *Drink Less; Live Better* will be a best-seller!"

Alex McRobert – The Mindful Life Practice

"It can sometimes take one person to plant a seed in your mind to act as a catalyst for making a change that you know will be for the better and for me Sarah has been that person. From following her own journey of taking back control, she represented that shift I needed to make for myself. The exhilaration I feel from the physical, emotional and mental benefits of giving up alcohol have felt so empowering – I have Sarah to thank for the steady, non-judgemental and honest support, which gave me the inspiration and determination to confront my relationship with alcohol head on."

DH – Client

"It's no surprise that Sarah would write a book that's loaded with just the right combination of compassion, kindness and sincerity to help those of us who are interested in changing our relationship with alcohol. Without judgement, she asks those questions we are often avoiding – the type of inquiries that trigger deep self-reflection or just enough introspection to make a small adjustment that reaps huge rewards. I love the way she weaves her story throughout the book while sharing the tips and tricks that paved the way for her alcohol-free journey. She's helped me to realise there's no one-size-fits-all answer to the question of how much or how little alcohol is right for me. While I suspect sober is where I'll end up, soberish is sometimes part of my journey and that's OK."

MB – Client

"I saw Sarah speak at the Mind, Body and Spirit Festival London and was blown away. Her words were kind, funny and insightful, more importantly she was infectious. Her message was clear: you can still have fun without the booze. Her story will be familiar to many, as it was me. For the first time, I felt empowered in my sober curious journey – ideas to beat inaction, support to make a start and joy over judgement. I'm so grateful her guidance has been part of my journey."

GA

Sarah Williamson

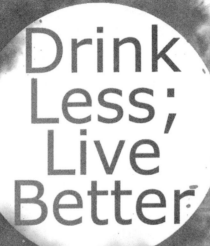

Drink Less; Live Better

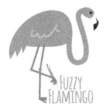

FUZZY
FLAMINGO

First published in 2023 by Fuzzy Flamingo
Copyright © Sarah Williamson 2023

Sarah Williamson has asserted her right to be identified as the author of this Work in accordance with the Copyright, Designs and Patents Act 1988.

ISBN: 978-1-7393669-4-0

Editing and design by Fuzzy Flamingo
www.fuzzyflamingo.co.uk

A catalogue for this book is available from the British Library.

The hardest bit about writing a book?
NOT the 50,000 words required on the page.
It turns out it's writing the dedication!

This book is...
For YOU walking the road less travelled.
For my fellow rebels, outliers and revolutionaries.
For each of us making an unconventional choice to be free
from one thing holding us back.
We move forward together.

Contents

PART 2: ACCEPTANCE 51

PART 3: ACTION   **111**

Introduction

I wrote this book with the hope it would help someone who was in the same position I was several years ago.

Someone who:

- Knew alcohol was taking more than it was giving but didn't know how to approach the situation.
- Was tired of the merry-go-round of feeling a bit low and using alcohol to add a bit of fun, but was scared of being miserable, lonely and/or boring.
- Understood all the ideas behind movement, rest and good nutrition, but was struggling to start or maintain them.
- Wanted to prove to themselves they were capable of more but was also afraid of finding it hard.
- Had a feeling that there was more purpose and passion to be squeezed out of their precious life but knew it was probably going to take some work to find out what.

I hope the wisdom and insights between these pages feel relevant to you, I trust you sense the feeling of love interwoven between the lines and I wish you the courage to make your next bold move.

Sarah

Coach and Chief of Belief at *Drink Less; Live Better*

www.drinklesslivebetter.com

PS. I believe in you

About Sarah

Sarah decided to execute a life experiment in which she went alcohol-free for a year. She thought she'd return to drinking at the end of the experiment because her life would be miserable, lonely and/or boring without it. Turns out she was wrong about that.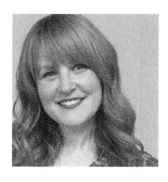

In this book, she shares some of her knowledge about choosing not to drink in a world where 'a drink' seems to be the answer to so many questions.

When she's not coaching her clients, creating her podcast, hosting retreats, speaking at staff well-being days or presenting at events and festivals, you are most likely to find Sarah walking in the Surrey Hills, drinking tea and eating cake or negotiating herself out of a tricky situation with a teenager!

This is a book of stories, insight, wisdom, strategies, resources and love. It takes you to the place where doubt and belief meet, where action follows and lasting change becomes yours.

PART 1

AWARENESS

"Awareness is the greatest agent for change."
Eckhart Tolle

CHAPTER

Why would you like
less/be alcohol-f

Well, here we are, let's start at the beginning.

I'm going to take a wild guess as to why you've picked up this book. I suspect you'd like to consider drinking less or becoming alcohol-free, perhaps you'd call yourself sober curious or maybe, just maybe, you've had enough hangovers, missing memories or bouts of low-level self-hatred after that 'one' relaxing drink. Perhaps a reconsideration of your relationship with alcohol might seem like a good idea right now?

Choosing to experiment with sobriety is about transformation.

First, we become aware of the change we want to consider, then we try some strategies to move ourselves closer to what we want. We might not get it right for a while, we may need different tools, plans and the support of others. Once we decide on a new path, it's still possible to make mistakes, of course, but we learn from them as we go. Let's not forget, if you continue to make the same choices, you're going to end up with the same results every time.

flawed and perfectly imperfect. We need to
the unhelpful patterns, behaviours and actions and
arn what thoughts, feelings and emotions are driving
them. When we are able to bring awareness to our patterns,
we then stand a chance to be able to change them.

One of the most important things to get straight in your
head before you decide to drink less or be alcohol-free for
a while is to get absolutely clear on the reasons WHY you
want that change. It's important because in those moments
when you doubt yourself you've got some ideas to go back
to and reassure yourself that you've made the right choice.

I'll tell you some of the reasons I chose to do my own
alcohol-free life experiment, but first a tip for you: once
you've figured out all the reasons why you want to drink
less or be alcohol-free, temporarily or permanently, write
them down on pieces of notepaper and put them in various
places where you'll see them regularly.

Here are some good places:

- In the front of your diary/notebook/planner.
- Inside a kitchen cupboard door.
- Used as a bookmark.
- Take a photo and save it to your favourites.
- Add to your phone notes app.
- Use it as a screen saver.
- Make a voice note of yourself reading it out loud.

Having your 'reasons why' noted in various places means
when you might be tempted to have a drink you can look
at them easily and use them as a tool to dissuade yourself

4

from any rubbish choices you were potentially about to make.

Here are the initial reasons why I decided to become alcohol-free for a while:

- I wanted to know if life would be as stressful, lonely or boring without alcohol as I'd led myself to believe.
- I wanted to know if it was possible to relax, connect with others and have fun without a drink, like I suspected it could be.
- The hangovers and brain fog were getting worse in my late thirties and early forties – I just couldn't get away with it like I had in my twenties.
- I wanted to be a more patient parent – no more selfishly rushing the kids through bedtime because I wanted to get back downstairs to my drink.
- I wanted to model something different for my children – relaxing in ways that are emotionally and physically healthier than I had been showing them.
- I wanted hangover-free weekends to enjoy my time away from work commitments.
- I wanted to maximise my nutritional choices – no more rubbish food choices dictated by low-level hangovers.
- I wanted to sleep deeply and wake up feeling as well as I could.
- I wanted to know I was giving myself the best chance of not getting breast, bowel, mouth, throat or liver cancer, dementia, high blood pressure, heart disease, liver disease or in any way compromising my immune system.

Allow yourself to be a beginner at this. We are going to move through this together, bringing awareness and acceptance to your past drinking behaviours and making an action plan for what's next. We'll then align your life to fit with what you value most.

ACTION POINT

Write down the reasons why you are going to choose to drink less or become alcohol-free for a while and save that list in various places.

A strong sense of purpose helps us move towards success. If you are able to get really clear on your 'WHYS' and then arrange your life around them for the next week or longer, you are much more likely to meet with success.

CHAPTER 2

Planning to take a break

Some people go straight into sobriety with an "I'll never drink again" goal and that is amazing and admirable.

Some people choose to work on a "one day at a time" basis.

There's no right or wrong answer in all of this. You need to choose whatever approach, goal, challenge, length of time is going to work for you. It's important that whatever length of break you choose, it feels GOOD, hopeful and optimistic. If it happens to feel a bit daunting, that's OK too.

I did things a little differently. I started with the idea of a break because that's what felt good to me. Not forever and not one day at a time.

I knew I could do a month alcohol-free – I had the evidence for that, as I'd completed successful Dry Januarys and Sober Octobers in the past. Doubling or tripling my goal to sixty or ninety days didn't seem challenging enough. I'm a sucker for a round number, so while 100 days sounded good to me, it still just didn't seem enough. I wanted to be able to question whether I could really do it.

In the same way people know they can run a 5k or a 10k

but start marathon training not knowing whether the final race is really achievable (congratulations to you if you've ever run a marathon), I picked 365 days! A year.

I decided a proper life experiment would be best if it involved all the big drinking activities in an annual social calendar. Christmas and all that season entails, New Year's Eve, my birthday, the races, pub lunches, family and friends' birthdays, a wedding, hectic times at work, festivals and holidays.

I was set to begin on 1st January 2020. I'd told myself that my nice round goal of one year should start on New Year's Day.

In preparation for my start date, I cut my drinking down significantly but I then began to wonder why I was waiting for January to start my virtual stopwatch. Who was I doing that for and why? Did I care about New Year resolutions? No, absolutely not. I've never seen a successful annual resolution through to the end of a year in my life!

If I was serious, why didn't I choose now?

If I could get through December 2019 without a drink, then it would give me the evidence that the whole of 2020 was possible, surely?

So, I started before I was ready.

In December, I went to a house party with some friends. I had a couple of G and Ts and we ate/played board games/danced and had fun.

The next morning, I woke up and knew that my life experiment had begun. I wasn't going to drink for 365 days from then.

Alcohol exploits ambiguity. I knew choosing a goal and really committing to it was going to be key to my early success.

ACTION POINT

1. Choose a date to start your challenge. Now flick forward in your diary to the date you plan to finish and make a note of it. As you flick through, make a mental note of any potential sticking points – we'll come back to talk about those, but for now, just 'see' them and don't be afraid!

2. Now, take a 'Day One Selfie' and save it… you'll want a record of the day you made this fabulous decision.

3. Write your goal down.

Your written goal will serve as a reminder. It's a way of bringing your vision into reality. Our ideas sometimes remain stuck in our minds until we write them down and commit to achieving them. Writing your commitment down will leave no room for misunderstanding. I'm keen on short-term goals. I enjoy having a clear marker in the future that I can aim for.

CHAPTER 3

Language is so important when choosing your drink less or alcohol-free goal

When we get sober curious and interested in our emotional and physical health and well-being, it's easy to fall into the trap of using someone else's language without first checking if it's a good fit for us. Do you like goals? Challenges? Resolutions? Intentions? What FEELS good for you?

I'd moved my start date forward from the 1st January into December and that was, in part, because I didn't want this to be a New Year's resolution. I also didn't want my year to be a goal or a challenge – these words feel to me like something to strive for or endure and, God knows, I cannot live in the strive or endure zone for longer than about twenty minutes, let alone a year… so what would be better? Hmmmm… a trial, a campaign, an undertaking, an experience…? Nope, not quite the right fit for me.

What about an adventure or a life experiment? Yep, either of those sounded like a good idea – it says medium term, full of possibility, potentially fun and stretching my comfort zone. I believe the way I chose my language around my 'alcohol-free life experiment' was fundamental to my early success.

Armed with the 'why', the 'plan' and the 'language' of a 365-day alcohol-free life experiment, I was ready to start.

The first time I had really known I was going to come to this point was in June 2017, but it took me two and a half years to be ready to move it forward. In that time, I struggled over and over with the ideas about why stopping drinking would be stressful, lonely or boring.

The second decision I made about my language was not to say, "I'm not drinking." Warning! A lot of what I'm about to say is semantics but hang in there!

"I choose to be alcohol-free as a little life experiment" sounds so much better to my brain than "I'm not drinking."

My brain likes the idea of a choice and prefers alcohol-free to not drinking (because I am drinking lots of other drinks). Adding in the reason why gives my brain a cute reminder every time I say it.

Even though my 365-day life experiment finished long ago, I continue to choose to be alcohol-free years later.

I cannot see myself ever saying I'm never drinking again because my brain got used to that being a lie all the times I said it between the ages of sixteen and forty.

ACTION POINT

Right now, it's so important for you to know why you want this break from alcohol, how long you want to do it for and what wording sounds good to you.

This next bit of your life is supposed to feel empowering, interesting and worthwhile – go into it feeling like it's a positive choice. PLEASE.

CHAPTER 4

What type of drinker are you?

I wouldn't have put myself into any one category of drinker when I was drinking. I drank in different ways, for different reasons, at different points in my life. At various times over the past thirty years, I was one (or more) of these:

- Emotional drinker: I drank to ease the discomfort of a particular feeling or to enhance an already elevated feeling.
- Social drinker: I drank because everyone else did.
- Weekend drinker: I drank because that's one of the things weekends are good for.
- Binge drinker: I drank because Friday nights out with the girls required it.
- Daily drinker: I drank to 'change gears' between day and evening.
- De-stress drinker: I drank to unwind and relax at the end of the day.
- Absent-minded drinker: I drank out of habit and not pausing to think of a better alternative.
- Evening out drinker and at home drinker: I drank because it's both what I did when I was out and what I did when I was at home!

- Celebratory drinker: I drank because all celebrations required it.
- Commiseration drinker: I drank because if something is already sad, it required making sadder.

In short, I drank for all the reasons and no reason at all.

ACTION POINT

Take a moment to consider the reasons you currently drink.

Chapter 5

It's all about what you gain, not what you give up

Once you have decided on your drink less or alcohol-free life experiment/challenge/goal, how will you frame it positively? I've talked about being mindful of the language I used and one of my thoughts was that I would try not to use the phrase 'giving up' alcohol or 'giving up' drinking.

I wanted to put the most empowering spin on this decision I could. I wanted to think of what I was doing as joyful and life enhancing, and if I think about giving up, I think of deprivation and denial.

I didn't want to allow my brain to head off in the direction of *it's not fair*.

Let's look at what's to be gained.

The thing that happened for me very quickly was **much improved sleep**. The effects of a few drinks can take a couple of days to work out of your system and cutting it out completely led to a much better pattern of sleep. I no longer stirred in the night, didn't need to get up to go to the bathroom or have a glass of water and I started waking earlier and feeling better first thing in the morning. What a joy!

More level moods. I had no idea I was riding such emotional mood roller coasters. If I had a hangover or even low-level brain fog in the morning, I didn't feel great, and therefore the people closest to me felt the full force of it. I didn't speak kindly to myself, and I was a more anxious person because of it. I'm so glad to be rid of that creeping hangxiety now.

More energy. More sleep and feeling better about myself has given me so much more energy physically, emotionally and spiritually!

My **skin improved** drastically. I think this was for three reasons:

1. I stopped putting a toxin in my body.
2. I started to actually use the moisturisers in my bathroom cabinet instead of falling into bed too knackered to use them.
3. I was better hydrated as I started to drink plenty of water for the first time in my life.

Time. I hadn't realised what a time suck drinking was. The time from 5pm thinking about drinking: *What will I drink? Do I have what I want in the house? When can I open the bottle? How much shall I have?* Then, once I'd opened the bottle and after dinner was cooked, I did nothing else useful. Some might call it relaxing. I now call it dead time. And, of course, there's the wasted morning time, hitting snooze and then eventually getting on with your day in a slightly underwhelmed way. I see it as time not wasted, a mind not zoned out and I love that.

Productivity. Would I have had the get up and go to study, train and certify for a new career if I was still drinking? I suspect not. I wanted to change my life in significant ways and being alcohol-free has given me not only the energy and time but also the clarity and mindset to get on and do it in a way that feels aligned and natural.

My **nutrition choices** have significantly improved since I chose to be alcohol-free. I used to reach for the crisps and nuts with a G and T or a glass of wine and, if I had any hint of a hangover, my breakfast choices used to be, shall we say, less than ideal. It's a different story now – I'm not flawless on this front but I have left my snacking habits behind, and I tend to start each day with a more nutritious breakfast or brunch.

I am happy about how **relationships** are unfolding around me. Not just with my family and friends but also new people in my life who are turning out to be a total joy.

Finally, **money**. How much cash did I waste over the years, not only on booze itself, but also taxis, carb-laden hangover cures, coffees and paracetamol. No more, my friends, no more.

I wouldn't ever have told you I spent too much on booze because what I was spending money on was fun, and hey, what price can you put on fun?

Now, I look back on situations that were supposed to be fun – big birthdays or parties, days at the races and other days out, weddings and anniversaries – I can remember very little as alcohol stole those memories.

I had my nights out drinking but also my nights in

drinking. This alcohol was just added casually to the weekly shop, of course, so it never really felt like spending money, but it was. My average weekly shop cost has since gone down significantly.

When I drank at home, I was also prone to a bit of late-night online shopping. It was often a surprise to see what urgent purchase on a Friday or Saturday night turned up on a Tuesday morning.

When I went out for dinner with friends, the dining element might have been £20/£30/£40 per head but the bill split was always for much more. We drank cocktails, fizz and wine all evening. When I'm out with my friends now, they always insist on taking the booze off the bill, so I don't pay for it. I'm really delighted to be out having a fab time, but I do feel good spending a fraction of the cash on a night out.

A while into my alcohol-free life experiment, I committed to doing something totally fabulous! I pay for a cleaner on a Friday, which fills my heart with joy! I never used to love cleaning and with the thought of choosing either a lovely clean house or a few bottles of booze – I choose a clean house every time!

When I finish work on a Friday and the kids get home from school, I have a quick scan of the room I'm in and think, *oh, my house feels lovely – I'm so lucky to have someone help me with this. I've chosen this for myself, and this is how I want Friday evenings to feel.*

ACTION POINT

Write your two lists. What am I gaining? What am I giving up?

CHAPTER 6

Feelings and emotions

I've heard it said before that one of the BEST things about being alcohol-free is feeling your feelings and one of the WORST things about being alcohol-free is feeling your feelings.

One of the first things I noticed when I decided to try my alcohol-free life experiment was how much more level and steady I felt. There was no longer any low-level brain fog or creeping anxiety, no more rising panic or feelings of unease. My mood was certainly helped by the fact that I was suddenly sleeping much more soundly and for longer due to the fact my body wasn't having to process all the toxins in alcohol.

I took a while to get used to the feelings of tiredness at the end of each day. When I was still drinking, I would look forward to a drink in the evening as a way of coping with being tired. I now realise that a drink did nothing to help with that feeling and indeed only exacerbated it. I had to look for other tools to help with the emotional tiredness. I chose to make time for going for a brief walk, having a bath, sitting down with a book or listening to a podcast. The feelings that I felt and naturally occur in most of our lives like tiredness, frustration and overwhelm needed slightly different tools to handle them, but one idea that I began to use regularly was taking the time to recognise the feelings and acknowledge them. Previously, I had been quick to pour a G and T or a glass of wine when I was overwhelmed. I felt guilty about whether I had the balance right between my work, family and the rest of my life. I was sad about some health issues within my family and this grief was never made better with alcohol.

I reconsidered how I could change things. Choosing to be alcohol-free has given me the chance to really think about how I want to feel in various situations in my life and the knock-on effect has been a positive impact on my behaviour both towards myself and others.

Inside my head is a much nicer place to be now. I no longer have huge internal arguments with myself about whether I can have a drink tonight, how many I can have, what time I can start or whether a white wine spritzer counts as a soft drink! My internal dialogue more often sounds like a kind friend rather than a critical enemy. I'm kinder, more compassionate and forgiving both towards myself and other people.

I find it easier to process my emotions and move on or to make a decision to think more deeply about them – where did they come from and why – what can I learn here? I don't punish myself for past mistakes 'drinking me' made. I'm more honest with myself, I acknowledge and accept the feelings that come and I know I'm better placed to identify them without alcohol than I ever was with a bottle of Pinot Grigio inside me.

Emotions – they are part of what life is, they come and go. It's common to experience a range of emotions in a day, an hour or even a few minutes and that's OK.

ACTION POINT

Make some notes about who, when, where and why you are in the habit of drinking. Is it every day at 6pm as you start to cook? Friday nights once the kids are in bed? Curry nights out with your partner? Sunday lunch round at your in-laws? Make notes so you can start to put a plan in place as to how you will tackle these flashpoints.

What alcohol do you have in your house right now? Can you resist it? If not, chuck it, put it in the loft or take it round to a friend's house for them to look after for the duration of the challenge. Do NOT leave it in temptation's way if you think it might whisper to you!

CHAPTER 7

Are you making this complicated?

I used to love a to-do list. I didn't have a structured way of keeping all my tasks in one place, but I tried to keep on top of where the heck I was with frantic list writing, keeping, doing and ticking.

A couple of years ago, I was working multiple part-time jobs – one job took up the majority of my time and I also had a small part-time contract, four freelance jobs and was trustee of a charity.

Why?

Well, people kept asking me and I didn't like to say no.

It served its purpose at the time. I liked the money and I liked being busy... oh, the joy of busy, I thought. I wore it like a badge of honour, as many people do.

I used to think that saying "If you want something doing, ask a busy person" was funny and correct – not any more.

I realise I was using busy as a way of keeping myself distracted, a way of not addressing the bits of my life that needed some time and attention spent on them – if I was busy crossing stuff off my list then I couldn't possibly have the time or head space to do anything else.

Besides – If I had written "address Friday night

23

collapsing on sofa with a glass or three of wine" on my list, that couldn't have been neatly ticked off.

It was a bit messy, it needed head space, it needed thinking about, it needed discussing with people who might try and reassure me I didn't have a problem... or did it?

Perhaps, I was avoiding the issue and I just needed to put a plan in place and do it.

I now know for sure that if I am questioning 'do I have a problem here?' then I almost certainly do. And that's all I need to know to then get on and make a change. Of course, it could be about pretty much anything – exercise, making time to relax, eating well, etc.

I was making everything a little bit complicated, and I was cluttering my mind. I don't like physical clutter around me, and I don't like mental clutter either – perhaps that was why I had to be a list keeper so that the detail was out of my head and on paper.

While I'm talking about pieces of paper... have you heard of Eisenhower's Matrix? I was introduced to this productivity tool and it really helped me to prioritise the tasks that were important and urgent and to also see that some tasks could be delegated or even eliminated. I do still allow myself to get over busy from time to time and the state of my desk is a really good indicator of my inner feelings. Once I have got my desk straight and prioritised, and my top couple of tasks for the day nailed down, I can move on much more easily.

I was always guilty of thinking I could fit much more

into my day than I realistically could, and it often left me feeling unaccomplished at the end of the working day – another reason why I used to have a glass of wine – the feeling of dissatisfaction was real and needed taking down a peg or three!

Here is what I didn't need to have when I decided to try my alcohol-free experiment:

1. Permission from anyone else.
2. Additional items on my mental to-do list, i.e. 'I must also cut out sugar'.
3. A set of commitments to other people I didn't want to fulfil.

And here is what I did need:

1. Belief in myself.
2. One short-term goal (not to have an alcoholic drink).
3. A diary with things in it that felt good and not at all overwhelming.

In summary, don't make your mission to try an alcohol-free life experiment complicated – keep it simple. Ask for support where you need it most.

Once I had my alcohol-free life experiment safely underway, I took the opportunity to begin to address other areas in my life that felt overwhelming, and I was able to streamline my head space too!

What a joy! I'm a work in progress, like everyone else, but calmer than I was before.

ACTION POINT

Eisenhower's Matrix:

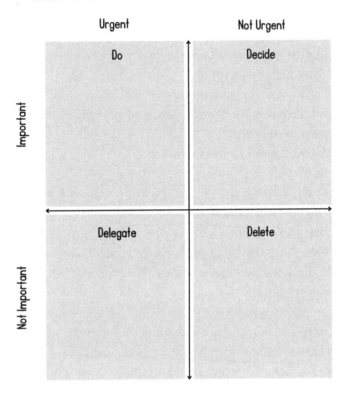

www.drinklesslivebetter.com

I use Eisenhower's Matrix to help me identify what really MUST be done in a given week, what can be given time and energy when I have it, what can be delegated and WHAT NEEDS TO GO!

CHAPTER 8

People pleasing

Drinking alcohol was sometimes something I did to please other people.

It's true, and isn't it odd?

There were a whole load of different reasons why I felt fearful about choosing my alcohol-free life experiment, ranging from the completely ridiculous to the just about justifiable.

One of the recurring themes, though, was worrying about what other people would say to me, say behind my back or say under their breath. Now, before we go any further with this, let's just explore the 'other people' concept. Who are the other people that I was worried about?

Well, inside my head, they are family, friends, colleagues, acquaintances, parents of my kids' friends, online pals and, in fact, also people I don't know. They exist in a kind of hierarchy in my mind, and I worried about what all the people would think when I told them I wasn't drinking for a whole year.

I now realise:

1. We always think that other people are more interested

in us and our lives than they actually are. This is normal and I have a word with my ego any time I start to think differently from this.

2. What other people think about us and say about us is none of our business and it should stay this way.

On my list of people, I was worrying about some of them I would never need to tell. I didn't owe them any part of my story. I needed to tell them I didn't drink as much as I needed to tell them I prefer DMs over trainers. It is information that doesn't matter to anyone who doesn't know you well.

Then I remembered another saying: "Those who matter don't mind and those who mind don't matter," and I absolutely knew that would be true with all my close family and friends. My husband barely batted an eyelid when I told him about my alcohol-free choice… and, let me tell you, he can be deeply cynical at times. Recently I told him I was going open water swimming for the first time, and he said, "Why are you doing that? You can barely swim the length of yourself!"

I love him but sometimes he is a little too honest!

(NB it turned out he was right to be cynical, I went once and have not been again since!)

So, my husband, family and friends either did or didn't comment, did or didn't want to chat about my choice, perhaps chatted behind my back or, of course, they thought nothing of it.

I struggled a bit with everyone else in my social circle.

I found myself over-explaining to colleagues, oversharing on a mums' night out and justifying my choice to a waitress in a bar!

And why?

Maybe because I like to people please. Saying yes comes so naturally to me. I had these ridiculous thoughts that turning down a G and T at a leaving party felt unsociable, saying no to fizz at a birthday felt rude and that replying that I'd prefer a soft drink at the races was not playing the hospitality game correctly.

I didn't want anyone else to feel uncomfortable. I was in discomfort myself and didn't want to share it. I didn't want anyone to have to make a special effort for me and I didn't want a light shone on my choice or anyone to ask me any questions about it.

BUT...

This has all been a gift of a lesson. With the passing of time, I've become so much more practised and therefore better at saying no to the offer of an alcoholic drink without fear of upsetting anyone.

People displeasing has become so much easier (and, of course, no one is really displeased – that was all my own interpretation of a situation that simply only existed in my overworked mind and not reality).

Being alcohol-free has allowed me to stop worrying so much what others think in all areas of my life and I am crystal clear about the fact that my choices are about me and not about anyone else – and I'm pleased about that. I'm really pleased.

ACTION POINT

Where does your people pleasing energy go at the moment?

Would you like to begin to change this way of behaving in the future? How can you start?

CHAPTER 9

Grey area drinking

How I found myself in the place known as 'grey area drinking'.

Now, I'm not really one for a label, a title or a neat little box, and if you'd have tried to put that label on me while I was still drinking, I'd have dismissed you straight away, either politely or not.

The passing of time is a wonderful thing, however, and I look back and can now clearly see that I was, for a very long time, a grey area drinker.

A grey area drinker is someone who falls into the bracket between never drinking and physical alcohol dependency. Society tends to view problematic drinking in black and white terms: you're an alcoholic and you need to be fixed or you're not an alcoholic and are therefore OK. Well, I think it's more nuanced than that. There's a spectrum between the extremes of rock bottom and every now and again drinking and it's a long spectrum.

A grey area drinker could be consuming a couple of glasses of wine each evening, someone who binge drinks at the weekend or someone who can abstain for a month at a time to prove they haven't got a problem. I was capable of any of those behaviours and, looking back, I fitted the description of a grey area drinker very neatly. I was never physically dependent on alcohol, but I used it to help me to alter my state of mind into relaxation/fun on a regular basis.

This can be a really confusing place to be when you first start to see alcohol for what it is. I'd say, "But I'm not doing anyone any harm. I'm sinking a couple of glasses of wine on the sofa and then I'm going to bed – what's the problem with that?" Ah… past Sarah… let me tell you the ways! But past Sarah wouldn't have listened to a word future Sarah had to say on the subject because she wasn't ready!

In the past, I moved along the grey scale – different ages, different friendship groups, different jobs, different circumstances, different seasons and different living arrangements all led to different drinking patterns. Apart from the periods in my life where I was pregnant or breastfeeding, I didn't ever choose to have a really extended time (more than thirty days) away from alcohol.

What I came to realise was that the more I moved along the grey scale, the more or less colourful other areas of my life became. If my joy was a rainbow, the vibrancy of that rainbow either faded or shone brightly depending on how much I was drinking.

I stopped myself from making a change around my drinking for a long time as I didn't want anyone to define me as having a problem.

The movies would have you believe that the end of your drinking career needs to be very dramatic with a family intervention and a massive rock bottom, but this doesn't need to be the case.

What if you chose for your drinking days to end with a quiet fizzle out instead of a big firework or massive drama? That's how it was for me. My grey area drinking changed shades of grey over a couple of years and, by the time I was ready to try my alcohol-free life experiment, I was moderating my drinking and never drinking more than two drinks at one time. However, the shades of grey no longer felt good, I wanted a full-on technicolour rainbow and I knew that to get one I had to do away with the other – so I did. Those grey clouds parted and, one by one, all the other areas in my life that had up until then been a bit less than joyful started to shine a bit brighter.

ACTION POINT

Rock bottom, a quiet fizzle out or a firm line in the sand? You choose.

CHAPTER 10

Self-judgement

I didn't want to stop drinking because I thought it would show other people I 'had a problem' and I assumed that if someone else wasn't drinking (without what I deemed to be 'a good reason') they had a problem too! Now I know better, I do better!

I used to be a total idiot about anyone who wasn't drinking, both behind their back and to their face, offering up really useful gems such as, "Go on, you could just have one," "It'll be more fun if you drink," and, "If you have some soda in your white wine it becomes a soft drink." Of course, this says everything about *me* then and nothing about *them*.

I couldn't fathom why or how people went out to a party or other night out and didn't drink, and I couldn't understand because I had no frame of reference for it myself – I'd never done it unless I was on antibiotics, pregnant, breastfeeding or driving – I mean, those are surely the only reasons you wouldn't drink, right?

Wrong – obviously!

People now ask me from time to time why I'm not drinking, and I see it as payback – or karma, if you will.

Because I've been that person, I know what to do with that question. I'm always happy to say I just feel better in life overall when I'm not drinking. I don't make a big issue out of it.

I have a friend who has never drunk and when we were chatting recently, she said I always wanted to know how she did it because she could see deep down it's what I wanted too – she's definitely right, and I'm eternally gratefully she never shut me down when I was being a pain! I was recognising something in myself that I wasn't comfortable with. Seeing other people drunk gives me fleeting moments of unhappiness now – I recognise past me drunk. I judge the parts of me I didn't like about myself. I understand the other person is me, a reflection of the parts of me I'm not so keen on. This is uncomfortable and something I take the time to think about whenever it happens. I try to change my self-judgement focus to compassion, and this helps me to soothe those awkward emotions.

Ah, yes – that was me then and now it isn't me. I'm much more loving towards myself now.

ACTION POINT

Go easy on yourself. Treat yourself as you would your best friend.

Let go of your need for anyone else's approval – *your* approval is what matters.

CHAPTER 11

Start dates don't matter – starting does

In January, when people start talking about detoxes, diets and not drinking for a month, I remember how I used to think about alcohol in the New Year and engaging (or not) in a dry month.

I can remember once claiming I was doing it Monday to Thursday, once that I was doing it as 'not drinking at home' and once I just made it through the first week before giving up. My birthday is the 4th of January, and I went through many years of telling all my friends that detoxes, diets and not drinking couldn't start until the 5th. I look back on my old self and wonder what I was trying to achieve with that. Was it a last-ditch attempt to hang on to the old party girl me? I don't know.

A month without alcohol gives us a physical break, it potentially stops a pattern of regular drinking and emotionally we get a chance to recalibrate without using alcohol to either cheer us up or numb us down. And that's all OK, isn't it?

Come February, I used to go back to my usual drinking ways. "I've had a month off booze. I've proved to myself and everyone else I don't have a problem with alcohol, so back to it."

I'd also use similar phrases in December. "I'm having a month off booze in January, so I can drink all the drinks in the run-up to Christmas and New Year, woohoo, go me!"

What if you go into January thinking you can do it and yet find you can't? Who will be there to hold your hand? What if you are overcome by guilt and shame because you didn't achieve what you set out to do? Will you laugh it off, like I did? Or will you beat yourself up in private, like I did too? Will you wonder why it was so hard? We will see those around us who were tripped up by unexpected events, either good or bad, when they felt they needed a drink to celebrate or commiserate, and those who couldn't get started in the first place.

January is a rubbish month for piling too much onto our to-do lists. Let's go into every New Year being kind and gentle on ourselves.

ACTION POINT

Are you ready to claim your start date?

Chapter 12

The place where doubt, belief and action meet...

One of my really good friends asked me a question recently when we were talking about change. Well, actually, we were having a brilliant conversation about values, but I'll address that in Part 4 ALIGNMENT. We were momentarily talking about change, and she asked me, "How do you do it? How do you get the agency to change?"

I flippantly replied, "Well, I think I just decide, and then I do it."

Then I paused. Hmm... there is actually more to it than that.

We started to draw ourselves some spidergrams because that's what we had just been doing when we were playing around with our values conversation (I know, I'm so lucky, my friends and I love having these life-affirming conversations)! I wrote 'action' in the middle. Action felt like a good starting word.

Action is where the outward change happened for me. However, the change had been happening inside my head for a considerable time prior to that.

I had spent a lot of time thinking about the action I was

going to take and there had been a long period of doubt before that.

Can I do this? Do I need to do this? Do I even really want to do this? I'm not that bad. I've not hit rock bottom. I'm probably fine, really.

My thought process went through a protracted time of adjustment, readjustment, checking out my feelings related to my thoughts, following through on new behaviours I wanted and reconsidering behaviours I kept slipping back into.

Somewhere along the line, I got hopeful, I started to believe in myself. I sensed change really was possible. I saw people who had some of what I wanted, and I endlessly copied them. I consciously chose new behaviours, and even more consciously left old ones behind and moved forward. I aimed for progress, not perfection. When I couldn't be kind to myself, I sought out others who could be kind to me, who believed in me. I made a goddamn massive effort. I practically made my change my full-time job for a while, I threw the kitchen sink at it. If something worked, I applied more of it. And if it didn't, I left it to one side. To be successful, to get the agency to change I wanted, I learned, I invented my own little process, a system, a framework. I took those early glimmers of hope and belief and acted on them. We could apply all of this to anything: changing our drinking habits, fitting in exercise, eating a more nutritious diet.

ACTION POINT

The distance, the gap, the space in between your dream and your reality is called action.

Can you identify three small actions that could start to move you in the direction of your dream?

CHAPTER 13

Excuses, excuses

My excuses were many and varied. What it really boils down to, though, I think, is a case of being stuck because you have a fear of trusting yourself, and a lack of clarity around what you really, really want for yourself in the short term, the medium term and the long term. Definitely, in my first summer sober, I had all of the excuses around festivals, weddings, barbecues, pub gardens and my reasons were based around the fear of not trusting myself and also what other people were going to say. I knew that if I gave myself the tiniest, tiniest window of opportunity not to stick with the goal that I'd set myself, it was all over and it would have been all over before it really began if I didn't stick clearly to my guns.

To get clear on what you want, it might be best to think about the bigger picture first. Who is the person you're becoming as far as your family is concerned, your work is concerned, your finances are concerned? There are so many different areas in life where alcohol has a massive impact. If that's too big for you, roll it back a bit. What are you looking for yourself in the next year or so? And if that's too much, then bring it right down into the present moment. What are you looking to get out of this week in your life or even this day? How can you make your life better this week without alcohol in it? Do you have a history of things not working out? Are you the person like me who said a million times before "I'm never drinking again" and that worked really, really well for as long as the hangover lasted?

For me, "I'm never drinking again" was said as a joke at the end of my drinking days. Absolutely nobody believed me when I said it out loud and, of course, I didn't believe it myself either. Until the moment where I really, really did mean it and that moment was when I got totally clear on what I wanted. My original idea was to be alcohol-free for a year – a massive stretch. I knew I could almost certainly do a month alcohol-free. I thought that if I could do a month, I could probably do something like three months, but I had no idea whether that year-long experiment was going to be achievable. However, I have got a history of things working out in my life when I take bold action. I use the evidence of knowing that I had met my husband at a particular point in my life and that it worked out amazingly. I've had children in my life when it worked out really beautifully. Mostly the right jobs have crossed my path in the moments that I've been looking for them and really, really wanting them. I refer to my history, looking at where things worked out well, and applying some of that learning to my year of being alcohol-free. I knew that if I focused on the smaller goals, the bigger goal would become available to me if I left it alone for now. That clarity about one year alcohol-free was broken down into smaller steps. And through that first summer sober, I was able to see each event as a stepping stone to the next one. Once I'd enjoyed an alcohol-free wedding, I knew in my heart I'd be able to do an alcohol-free festival. Once I'd got through an alcohol-free festival, pub gardens were going to be an absolute walk in the park, or a picnic in the park that often used to be boozy affairs and no longer are for me. Getting totally clear and then trusting yourself helps you to see those excuses for what they really are, helps you to put those excuses aside and say, "These are not my stories, this is not who I am, I'm clear about what I want and I totally trust myself to go for it."

If you can't 100% trust yourself at the moment, who are the people you can gather around you? Who will be able to cheer you on? Who will be able to hold you accountable? Who do you need to share your story with so that they understand how much this means to you? Let's take those excuses apart. Let's get clear and let's face that fear of trusting yourself.

ACTION POINT

Who are your potential cheerleaders or accountability partners? Would it feel good to ask them for support?

CHAPTER 14

Alcohol as a gift

I was that person who gifted alcohol all the time. To a friend when I went round for dinner, to a sports coach for helping my kids, to a teacher for seeing through another school year, to a colleague for a birthday, to a family member at a party or anniversary, to a… hang on, this list could be long and repetitive. I gifted alcohol to most people for most reasons and I didn't think anything of it. It's an entirely socially acceptable gift, it's normal, it's thoughtful, it's nice. Oh! But is it?

You see, I've changed my mind about alcohol. For all the many, many years I drank, I gifted the gift I'd have been most pleased to receive myself – a bottle of wine or fizz. Every time I bought a bottle for a friend, I made sure I was choosing something I knew I'd seen them drink before or that I was fairly certain they'd like, but when I was choosing for someone who'd helped my kids or was an acquaintance, rather than a friend, I just guessed at what they liked but never considered the fact that they might not drink. No one ever handed me back a present and said, "No thanks." And why would they? We are taught to accept a gift and be grateful, aren't we?

I bought this booze for other people because in my drinking years it's what I would've wanted as a gift – it's easy and it's thoughtless.

Now, I try to put a bit more energy into gift giving. I try to learn a bit more about the person if I don't know them well – I try to buy gifts that will be happily received.

I happen to be someone who doesn't particularly love things, items, stuff that needs a home in my house. I happen to love dispensable gifts, things that you use and then are finished with – so I tend to now focus on that idea for others. As a side note, alcohol used to fit brilliantly into the dispensable category – drink it and recycle the bottle.

Now I love to receive and give fresh flowers or small plants for the garden, book vouchers, lovely hand or body lotions, delicious chocolates, homemade goodies or nice notebooks. A bit more thoughtful and some effort required, but I feel so much better about not buying all that wine now I'm not drinking it.

I was recently given two bottles of fizz as a thank you for something I did for a neighbour, which I gratefully accepted (I didn't want to appear rude) and I've added it to a box in my shed with a number of other bottles people have given me. They sit there because they are lost in no man's land. I wouldn't drink them, I'm unlikely to gift them on… I suppose a guest might want a glass in the future… I don't know! They could be headed for the kitchen drain at some point – I feel no sorrow about that idea, they are just clutter taking up shed space, really.

When I first went alcohol-free, I had no problem at all

pouring all those half bottles of spirits down the sink – I watched it drain away, thinking how glad I was that my body wasn't consuming those empty calories and toxins. Why would I ever gift anyone else a hangover when I don't want one myself?

This is my gift, my act of kindness to my friends and family – no more alcohol as gifts!

ACTION POINT

Repeat after me: "I do solemnly swear I will no longer buy alcohol as a gift – I can do better than that!"

CHAPTER 15

Small words, big impact

I love thinking about words, changing words, adding words in or emphasising words to be able to see or, more importantly perhaps, hear big differences in my language. Here's an example of one of my all-time favourite word changes.

"I'm loving living my sober life but sometimes I feel like I might be missing out." The question to myself is why does there have to be a 'but' in that sentence? My desire for an amazing sober life doesn't negate my feelings of FOMO from time to time.

"I'm loving my sober life and sometimes I feel like I might be missing out." This makes room for both emotions; changing from 'but' to 'and', I can shift my focus from conflict to resolution. No more: "What do I do? Poor me." Instead, what's my FOMO driven by? How can I create the fun times I want with the people I really love?

One word change from 'but' to 'and' can make a massive difference. 'But' often closes a dialogue, whereas 'and' allows for a curious question or reconsideration.

- "I know I want to stop drinking but it's hard" versus "I know I want to stop drinking and it might be hard."

- "I'd love to go to that event but I'm anxious" versus "I'd love to go to that event and I'm anxious."
- "I'd love to ask that person if I can join them, but I might get rejected" versus "I'd love to ask if I can join them, and I might get rejected."

The first part of the sentence represents something I want to do, it's an action in line with my values. The second part of the sentence represents my reasons for not wanting to engage in the action – of course, mostly fear based. I might understand something is hard and still want to try it. I can feel anxious and still go ahead and do it. I can get rejected and survive. Being told 'no' won't kill me.

- "I'd love to go to that event and I'm anxious."
- "I'd love to ask if I can join them and I might get rejected."

Both parts of these sentences are true now and they sound OK to me. They acknowledge my fears and help me to move forward.

That's one word change. What about if we add a small word in? My favourite for this is the word 'yet'. It's a growth mindset game changer. "I'm not sober," sounds a bit sad. "I'm not sober yet," sounds hopeful. The word 'yet' is powerful. It helps us to see learning as a journey, helps us to maintain engagement and increases our confidence when perhaps we feel out of our depth. Have a look at the work of Dr Carol Dweck. She is amazing, and her TED talk is fabulous.

So, that's a word changed, and a word added into a sentence. What about emphasising a word?

How often do you tell someone close to you that you love them? There's a teenager in the hallway about to leave the house. There's a partner hopping into the car to drive to work. There's a toddler being dropped at nursery. "Love you." I say it often. It is usually always heartfelt, usually well received and mostly replied to. "Love you," on the end of a phone conversation with a friend. "Love you!" shouted out of the car window to my mum and dad as I left their house. "Love you," to a colleague I adore at the end of a Zoom call. And then one day I realised a word was missing, a small word, a tiny word: 'I'. 'I' helps me to claim the sentence.

"I love you. I love you. I love you."

I've been taking hold of the power of that tiny, tiny word and I've been using it hard. My family hear a fuller sentence now, one that feels more meaningful and less added on as an afterthought, or casually thrown around, and, of course, it's coming back to me like that too.

"I love you."

ACTION POINT

Are you able to say "I love you" to those you care about most?

Are you able to say "I love you" to yourself?

Go on, do it now…

PART 2

ACCEPTANCE

*"The truth will set you free
but first it will piss you off."*
Gloria Steinem

CHAPTER 16

Will my drink less or alcohol-free life be too difficult?

When I first decided to become alcohol-free for a whole year, I thought there'd be blood, sweat and tears. I thought the task at hand would be hideous and hard work.

To my surprise, that didn't come to pass. There was no blood, sweat, or tears shed and here's the shocker – there was learning, connection, fun and joy!

As I started to drink less in preparation for going alcohol-free, I read books I didn't know existed from a genre called 'quit lit' and here you are today reading my version today. Thank you.

I believe these books mainly fall into two main types: science-y and memoir-y. Think about your mindset before you delve into the treasure trove of this section of the bookshelves and feed the part of your brain that needs either information or stories (or both).

These books really helped me to see alcohol through new eyes. I felt like I was able to understand why I had drunk in the way I had and how I could start to change. I bought some physical books but also downloaded some audiobooks to listen to while I walked my dog.

I then realised that there were podcasts on the subject and loved testing out which ones I loved most. Please check out the *Drink Less; Live Better* one – it's short and snappy, meant to be quick love notes to inform, inspire and share my story – but others out there are longer form and interview based. Go and search for what appeals to you.

Have you ever heard of habit tracker apps? I hadn't, but in the early days of my alcohol-free experiment, I used one to keep a track of the number of days I'd been alcohol-free, and I loved seeing the time add up. I always made sure I ticked that I hadn't drunk alcohol first thing in the morning so that my brain knew what my intention for the day was. There are loads of specific sober day counting apps – find one that suits you, or if the thought of counting sober days is off-putting for you then don't! If you prefer a low-tech way of life, then you might prefer to tick your dry days off on a calendar or in your diary.

Always do what feels best for you – you don't have to copy anyone else's version of alcohol-free unless it feels good to you. This drink less or alcohol-free journey is supposed to feel like a joyful, positive decision and not in any way a punishment.

In my early days of not drinking, it sometimes felt a bit like a full-time job – I put a lot of my energy into it. I took the time to read, listen and journal about the thoughts I was having. In prioritising the habit of not drinking, it became easier and easier because I put it at the forefront of my mind. I knew it was important and I was able to stack up week after week without a drink because I made it a non-negotiable. The more distance I put between my last drink and now, the better I feel in mind, body and soul.

The tools I used in the early days gave me ideas of how to talk to my friends about the choice I'd made, gave me hope that I could do what I set out to do and made me feel less lonely about my choice.

Will your alcohol-free life be too difficult? I don't think so. It's likely to be calmer and easier in so many different ways.

Remove whatever difficulties you can 'see'. When I first decided I was going to drink less, I happened to have a box of six bottles of rosé wine in my house – at the time this was one of my favourite things to drink. I took it round to my neighbours to store and then I only went and picked up a bottle if I was going to take it to a party or go round to a friend's house. This stopped me from drinking it at home. When that wine was gone, I didn't replace it.

The other alcohol that was in my house needed tackling. I poured it down the sink. I had to build up to doing it and I felt really odd pouring it away. There were random bottles of ouzo, limoncello, cherry brandy and other holiday purchases or gifts that were easier to pour away because I wasn't really emotionally attached to them, but the half bottle of gin or vodka I struggled to get rid of – perhaps it was because I didn't want to let go of the thought of not drinking them for a whole year, perhaps it was because it felt like a waste, perhaps it was because I liked the bottle labels, or a combination of reasons.

I had (more or less) come round to accepting that

alcohol was a toxin and wasn't helping my physical or emotional state, so I took a deep breath, poured them away and put the bottles out for recycling. Once I had done it, I felt a certain freedom. If those bottles weren't in my house, they weren't calling me to drink from them – I suppose I felt a bit safer.

The only alcohol that was left in the house from then on was my husband's beer and whiskey because these are drinks that have never appealed to me – I'm not at all tempted to want to drink them.

So, with the alcohol removed and a bit of a plan in place, life instantly felt a bit less 'difficult'. Are you ready to make your life a little bit less difficult?

ACTION POINT

Tips to make your drink less or alcohol-free life a bit easier:

- Books.
- Podcasts – Find the *Drink Less; Live Better* Podcast wherever you listen.
- Habit trackers – electronic or on paper.
- Get rid of any alcohol in the house.

CHAPTER 17

Drink less or alcohol-free?

I cut down my drinking before I decided to go alcohol-free. Sometimes I went stretches without drinking and occasionally I had a mad blowout, but each time I did it led me closer to stopping.

I didn't have a description for how I was changing my behaviour then, but I do now. If I could go back in time, I'd tell myself, "This is harm-reduction or sober-curiosity and this is a good pathway towards looking after your physical and emotional well-being." I was bringing awareness to my thoughts, feelings, behaviour and the results I was getting. I was challenging myself about what I believed. I was educating myself. I was lining myself up for success.

During my late thirties, I'd started to become uncomfortable about the way I drank but couldn't figure out what to do about it. In an average week at home, I didn't drink more than the UK government guidelines for 'safe' drinking limits in women, but when I went out with my girlfriends, I always drank more than I intended to and always had a hideous hangover the next day.

As far as the chief medical officer's guidelines are concerned, if women drink more than six units in a single sitting that is considered binge drinking. On average, one large glass of wine contains three units of alcohol, so I only needed to be drinking two large glasses of wine to be bingeing. I hate the word bingeing – it even sounds ugly! Bingeing is apparently what I was doing when out with the girls and the price I paid seemed to get heavier and heavier. I was feeling physically and emotionally exhausted.

In 2017, I had a night out with some friends in London and the next day I suffered one of the worst hangovers I had ever had. I've kept the travel card from that night out in my purse ever since. I keep it as a reminder of how I never, ever want to feel again. The feelings of shame and guilt lasted well over a week, and I still have flashbacks that catch me out from time to time.

Through 2018 and 2019, the idea popped into my head every now and again that I should cut back my drinking on nights out. However, I never got round to actually cutting back – I just thought about it. I thought I had to behave the way I always had, as that was what was expected of me.

When I was ready to change, I started with changes I could make at home. I started buying really small single-serve bottles of wine so that I didn't feel the need to finish a full-sized bottle. They're more expensive per ml of alcohol but I knew I was benefitting my health massively by not drinking a whole bottle of wine, so I didn't care.

I then began to tell myself a new story about who I was on a night out. I would tell myself, *I am the person who goes to the pub with friends and enjoys two small glasses of wine and no more.*

This took me a while to perfect but, once I had it as a firmly entrenched belief about who I was, it worked a dream for me.

Drinking less over time was a massive part of my pathway to being able to choose alcohol-free for myself further down the line. I had a long time of moderating my drinking before I took the leap and went alcohol-free.

When I was cutting down the amount I was drinking, I had a very clear set of ideas about what I wanted the amounts to be. I needed these ideas so I had something to measure my alcohol consumption against. I needed to be able to decide whether I was being successful or not.

Drinking less might be a good choice for you if you are happy to learn from experiences and mistakes, you are happy to change your mind if things don't work out, you can rely on your ability to stop drinking after one or two drinks or you can see a future life for yourself where alcohol features.

Going alcohol-free might be a good choice for you if you feel like this is the break you need now, you like a straightforward and unambiguous decision, you cannot rely on your ability to stop drinking once you've started and you cannot see a place for alcohol in your future imagined life.

We should all choose what works best for us. Drinking less led me very neatly into alcohol-free, for other people a hard stop works well and for others getting their drinking to a place of moderation is their dream goal. Each to their own. No judgement here.

ACTION POINT

Are you currently considering drinking less, cutting back, reducing, moderating or thinking about a hard stop for a period of time or forever? Write a few notes to help you gain some clarity. Will you set yourself some parameters? How will you measure? How will you know if you are meeting with success?

CHAPTER 18

The liminal space

I spent several years undecided before I was ready to make my final choice about becoming alcohol-free for a year. I was in a place where I was back and forth, not quite ready to commit to the change. I hadn't realised there's an area between places, transient spaces, compartments, corridors, chrysalises where you move from one place to another, where the journey from A to B is made possible.

We cannot click our fingers and become different immediately. We need the opportunity to think, to learn, to grow and to develop and that can all happen in this space, the magical space called the liminal space. We might go into this messy middle ground with eyes wide open to the change that's happening. You may know nothing of it until you are out the other side or, indeed, you may never know you were in it at all.

The liminal space could apply to so many different life scenarios; becoming alcohol-free, changing careers, having children, choosing partners, deciding where to live, the 'in limbo', on the threshold feeling that comes with knowing you're stepping forward into something new. The liminal space is the middle bit, sometimes comfortable, sometimes not, the place of transition of neither here nor there, of uncomfortableness, questioning, not readiness. But looking back, it's where the magic happened for me. I felt as if I was poised, ready for something different, but not knowing if I was really bold enough or ready enough. What if I made the leap and failed?

Yes. What if? What if?

'What if' came up a lot. And we know and love that voice, don't we? It's sent from our brain to keep us safe, perhaps from thinking other people are judging us or misunderstanding us. I chose to see the liminal space I was in as a gathering and turning point. I asked myself questions. I thought long and hard and, when I was ready, I committed. I turned away from some old behaviours and accepted some new ways of being that I was sure were going to serve me better. Looking back, I was right, but I didn't know that at the time. I just made a choice. I drew a boundary and stepped forward out of the prison of indecision. I hadn't realised I'd been holding myself back until I chose to free myself. Of course, I was the only one holding myself back. No one else was responsible for that. While I was in the liminal space, I sought other people's opinions. I researched. I thought long and hard. I dismissed some feelings, challenged myself and came, eventually, to a point of acceptance. It was a time of growth that was, at times, horribly unpleasant. I saw some thoughts as truths when they weren't. I told myself stories that were founded on shaky ground, and I asked myself endless questions to find out the reality of my situation, both past and present.

I'm grateful now that I recognise the liminal space I was in and I recognised it while I was in it, too, although I wouldn't have called it that back at that time. What did I call it? I called it the place of stuckness. It was the messy middle. I called it this because I thought I was stuck. I felt I was stuck. I behaved as if I was stuck. Poor me!

I wasn't stuck. I was in between who I was then and who I am now. The place of stuckness was exactly where I needed to be then. Although, the liminal space does sound much better, and the place I am now is exactly where I need to be. If you're feeling a bit stuck, a bit in between, undecided, or untethered, try calling it the liminal space and find some comfort in the idea that you are moving in the perfect direction. There are brighter days ahead.

ACTION POINT

Can you think of some times in your life where you've been in limbo, stuck or in between situations? List them and then consider how you felt after you were through that time.

CHAPTER 19

I'm a human BE-ing
not a human DO-ing

I came to the realisation that I was sabotaging all my well-being activities. Through my late thirties and into my early forties, I was becoming more aware of the mind, body and soul connection. I was working full time, had two children, a husband, dog and all the other things a lot of people have in their lives, but I was feeling overwhelmed, and having a wind-down drink at the end of the day was one of the ways I chose to shut off emotionally.

I was getting more and more interested in personal growth and development. I was experimenting with life-enhancing practices like meditation and mindfulness. I'd become more committed to getting some exercise each week, either running, going to an exercise class or yoga. I'd taken more of an interest in my nutrition, using good quality supplements and making green smoothies each day.

I decided to increase positivity in my life in as many different ways as I could. I stopped watching or listening to the endlessly negative news, I curated my social media feeds to show me only inspiring people, I chose uplifting podcasts and audiobooks to listen to and hung out in real life with people who were radiators of warmth and love. All of this was amazing for my physical, emotional and spiritual well-being.

I was starting to feel like a grown-up but there was one thing that didn't feel right. I was adding more and more 'practices' in; getting up early in the morning to meditate, to journal, to be grateful. I was making time to exercise, I was choosing healthy menu plans and all of this 'adding things in' to my life was great, but…

I needed to take something OUT. And I didn't want to admit to it.

What's the point of meditating if you've got a bit of a hangover and can't concentrate properly?

What's the point of eating well if you are overconsuming toxins in your drinks?

What's the point in taking fancy supplements when you are drinking poison?

Why would I keep doing all these good things and not stop one of the really damaging things?

Around the time all this was going around in my head, I had a breakthrough thought and it was this:

I am a human BE-ing not a human DO-ing.

I wanted to stop feeling overwhelmed, so I started to cut commitments that didn't feel good, I only said yes to things that felt like a 'HELL YES' and I considered the needs of myself and my family before others. I prioritised exercise, nutrition and I took the time to be very still and very much a human *being*.

I bought myself a necklace with a bee on it to remind myself every day that I am concentrating on being a human *bee*-ing and that overwhelm is not my friend.

I no longer needed alcohol in my life – I didn't need to escape from anything any more. I recognised that and, from then on, I could start to do something about drinking less.

ACTION POINT

Do you have any do-ing activities you could start to spend less time on to make more time for be-ing?

CHAPTER 20

Making new friends
in your forties and beyond

In my twenties, I had old school friends with whom I'd bonded because of a shared educational or locational background and a love of drinking. I usually dated over a drink or two because… well… because I did, and it seemed as if everyone else did. After work activities and socialising always revolved around drinking.

In my thirties, I met a whole wave of new friends. We all had children in our mid/late twenties and early thirties, and bonded over playgroups, walks with the babies, tea or coffee round each others' houses and baby-centred groups (all of which we enjoyed as much for our children as for ourselves).

Meeting people who were sharing a similar experience to me was so important at that time.

I'm going to say that again and I'm going to come back to it in a minute:

Meeting people who were sharing a similar experience to me was so important at that time.

As my thirties were ticking along, I went back to work part time, my babies became toddlers and then school-age children, I shifted my work hours back to full time, we moved house and life was good. Better than that – brilliant, even.

I had everything from my wildest dreams – physical and emotional health, an amazing husband, two fabulous children, a supportive extended family, a lovely house in a beautiful town, a dog and job with a nice line manager and colleagues, money to pay the bills and go on holiday and lots of friends to spend time with.

While my daytime activities rarely revolved around drinking, my evening socialising always did. I was often the friend who organised the social activities and I don't think it ever occurred to me that I could organise fun that didn't involve dinner or a pub/bar – it was just the go-to activity. As I started to drink less, I asked my friends more often if they fancied a walk or brunch rather than an evening out and no one has ever said no. Yet. We do still go for nights out, but I am so happy to have alcohol-free drinks that I never care about what my friends are drinking.

So that brings me here. I'm in my forties now. I thought I'd already met most of my friends for life. I'm so lucky, I have university friends, old work colleagues, friends with kids the same age as mine and, of course, my husband. That's it, isn't it? That's all the friend boxes you need to tick?

Brilliant.

Almost everyone I know knows I'm not up for getting plastered. I'm a slightly improved version of myself – Me

Version 2.0, perhaps – and I haven't lost anyone who really mattered along the way.

But back to something I said earlier:

"Meeting people who were sharing a similar experience to me was so important at that time."

It was important when I was a new mum and had no idea what I was doing. It turned out to be important again when I was newly alcohol-free and, at times, I had no idea what I was doing or if this was really the right choice for me. I wanted to be bolstered by other people around me who have followed a similar thought process to me and decided that alcohol doesn't deserve a place in their lives right now. I want to have fun, laugh, talk about future goals and dreams (both mine and other people's), tell stories and share experiences.

I want to go out as Me Version 2.0 and know and love other people like me. I want to wake up hangover free and carry on a conversation where we left off, not struggle to piece together vague memories of last night.

The friendships I've made with other sober people over the last few years have been invaluable and are a rock-solid part of my life now.

I urge you to find your new sober people too – you won't ever regret it.

ACTION POINT

Which friendships are you putting energy into right now? Are they the right ones? Is there plenty of give and take in those friendships? Is there love or affection for each other? Do you come away from interactions feeling better than you did before?

CHAPTER 21

Does your drinking have an impact on your children?

Yes. I'm afraid so. Regardless of how old they are. (I know I wouldn't have wanted to hear this a while ago – so, sorry to deliver news you might not want.)

When my children were very small and after I'd stopped breastfeeding, I started using alcohol as a way of celebrating the end of the week. At the time, I would often happily not drink Sunday to Thursday but Friday nights became a ritual of over-drinking.

I look back now and wonder how this phase in my life got so out of control. I started binge drinking on a Friday night, using the reason that it was the end of the week and needed celebrating.

I would get together with a group of girlfriends who all had children of a similar age, we'd cook the kids' tea and then get stuck into the wine or fizz. We had a giggle, we chatted about what had gone on during the week, what our weekend plans were, what we wanted our futures to look like and, of course, we talked endlessly about our children.

We shared stories, experiences and dreams and bonded

because of the phase we were in in our lives. Of course, this could have been enough by itself, but it wasn't – we also bonded because we drank together.

Although we were thinking we were having meaningful conversations on a Friday night, they were rarely remembered the next morning and we were never able to pick up where we left off and continue. We probably had the same conversation every Friday night for years!

We would open a bottle at about 5pm and husbands would swing by from 7pm onwards to collect mums and toddlers and take them home. By this time, I would be totally done for. There were many Friday nights where I didn't cook for my husband and myself, I got the children into bed quickly (or he did) and then I either passed out on the sofa or went straight to bed.

A crushing hangover and two very early rising toddlers is surely a special kind of hell. Those Saturday mornings were not well spent. I cannot tell you how many times I watched *Thomas the Tank Engine* at 6am on a Saturday wondering if I was going to be sick or pass out – it was not good. I am not proud.

All of this was done in the name of fun and, at the time, I really did think it was fun, but I look back now and wonder why none of us questioned what we were doing – or if they did, I didn't hear it.

All of this came to a very natural end when the children got a bit bigger and Friday nights started to involve clubs after school or other activities.

Where I had been one of the instigators of the Friday

night fun, I started to offer to host it less and enjoy hangover-free mornings more.

When I first decided I'd go alcohol-free as a little life experiment, I wondered about the impact my drinking on Friday nights had had on my children. Obviously, I was not emotionally present for them on Friday evenings once I'd opened that first bottle.

Today I try not to dwell on decisions in my past I would now make differently. Today I focus on all the good stuff. I believe that a lot of parenting is about modelling behaviour and I now know my children are seeing and hearing about behaviours around alcohol that make me feel much more positive.

ACTION POINT

Have you ever stopped to consider the impact your drinking is having on the people you love most? If you haven't, I lovingly suggest now might be the time to do so.

CHAPTER 22

I'm alcohol-free but my partner isn't

I'm the only adult in my house who doesn't drink alcohol.

My husband drinks and I don't and that is OK with me – most of the time.

This whole alcohol-free thing has been a learning curve for everyone in our household. When I decided to do my year-long alcohol-free life experiment, my husband and I discussed it briefly before I started, and it seemed like no big deal for him. It was something I was doing, and he was going to be a bit of a bystander. I never expected him to be a cheerleader – I was making the choice for myself, and I didn't think I needed anyone else to tell me that I was doing a good thing or validate my choice in any way.

So, I chose to stop drinking and he carried on as he ever did.

Oh... screech of brakes a couple of weeks later... hang on a sec. What I hadn't articulated out loud (or indeed to myself) was the fact that my brain had assumed that when I stopped drinking my husband would notice my beautiful, technicolour, alcohol-free life and decide that he wanted all the good stuff and choose to stop drinking as well.

In my fantasy world, he'd say, "Oh, darling heart, I've noticed how radiant you look, how happy you are, what an amazing example you're setting for our kids, how much money you've saved and I want all of this too – I'm ditching the booze," and then we'd dance off into the moonlight to romantic music and congratulate ourselves on how clever we'd been to find this brave new world together.

Dear reader...

That is NOT what happened.

At the start of January 2020, I asked him if he fancied a dry January and he said, "No thanks." (In fact, it was ruder than that, but that was the gist.)

In the spring of 2020, I thought I would tell him all the benefits of being alcohol-free, so I wasn't keeping all the benefits a secret, and I expected him to then say to me, "Oh yes, the scales have fallen from my eyes. I didn't realise what I was missing but I do now, I'm going to join you."

But, no.

So, having suggested that he stop and he didn't, and then hoping he would stop without me mentioning it again and he didn't, I stopped giving it too much brain space.

My husband drinks a few beers on a Friday and Saturday night or whenever we go out together, he drinks when we socialise with friends and family and, every now and again, he gets blasted when he goes out with his friends.

I don't judge him – I used to do the same and more/worse.

I don't even wish it was different. A really important thing for me to remember is that I was unhappy with the way that drinking was making me feel and he isn't experiencing the same feelings as I had.

When he cracks open a beer on a Friday night, I make sure that I have a lovely drink at the same time, so it feels like we are still connecting over Friday night chill time. I'll have an alcohol-free G and T or a fancy-pants mocktail.

When we are in a bar together, I choose a ginger beer, a lime and soda or an AF lager.

Mostly, I stay in my own lane with my choice not to drink – I don't try to bring any friends or family over to my side of the street on the not drinking front.

I see my husband continuing to drink and I choose not to be affected by his decision.

He isn't alcohol-free and I am.

Together and apart, we are so much more than our drinking habits.

This might or might not be the case for you.

ACTION POINT

How do you feel about people drinking around you at the moment?

What makes you feel particularly uncomfortable and what can you cope with?

Chapter 23

Fixed mindset versus growth mindset

We want to feel like we're making progress, even if we're far from perfect right now. So, how can we do this? Have you heard of a fixed mindset versus growth mindset?

Someone with a fixed mindset believes their intelligence, talents and abilities are set qualities or traits and someone with a growth mindset understands that learning, practising and persistence can be developed.

Let's look at an example. Someone with a fixed mindset might say something like, "I'm unlucky, I'm not good at sport," and someone with a growth mindset might say something like, "I'm trying a few different sports to see which one I like best; I haven't yet found my passion."

Hmm. Hang on a sec. Did you catch the most important word in that last sentence? Yes, correct. YET.

'Yet' is such a beautiful word. In your moments of learning, practising and persisting, use the word 'yet'. I haven't learned this… yet. I cannot get the hang of this yet. This isn't sticking yet. All beautiful examples.

We're growing. We're seeing the possibility in our future. It's not our current reality, but we're heading towards our vision. Let's try some others:

- "I don't know how" versus "I can learn how."
- "I can't make this better" versus "I can find ways to improve."
- "I don't like challenges" versus "Challenges lead to growth."
- "Other people are better at this than me" versus "What can I learn from them?"

When we are motivated to embrace challenges or new 'ways of being', we risk possible failure, and avoiding a challenge prevents that possible failure. We might be trying to protect ourselves. Let's ask what's the worst that can happen? Is the answer so bad? Can you go ahead anyway? We can decide to accept that failures are part of our growth. Try to see them as temporary setbacks and perhaps even necessary in the pursuit of goals worth aiming for. Don't give up, setbacks might just turn out to be your stepping stones. Can you look around you and see other people's success as a source of inspiration? Don't feel any threat or jealousy. When you see someone else has a bit of what you'd like, know that's because somebody else is being, doing or having what you'd like... and you can be, do or have it too. They've just found a way that works for them.

Can you ask for help, support or feedback? See this as a part of your journey. Don't ever feel in any way 'less than' if you need a hand. In this life, we rise by lifting each other. Someone further ahead will have been where you are now and, hopefully, they will remember what it feels like and can offer you what you need to move forward.

Let's recap on what will help us.

1. Remove that fixed mindset inner voice. I cannot do this versus I cannot do this *yet*.
2. Know and believe that you can improve; our brains were designed to learn.
3. Practise and be persistent.
4. See setbacks as temporary, not a whole world of disaster. Use other people as a source of inspiration and support.

Let's just take a moment to recognise, as in many areas of life, that this isn't black and white. We tend not to be 100% fixed or 100% growth-minded; of course, we're a mix of both. I'd urge you to straighten your back, wiggle your shoulders down a bit and remember the magic word YET. Next time you're feeling a bit stuck, it's just possible it'll get you moving along your path another step or two. If we're heading in the right direction of our dreams, that can only be a good thing, can't it?

ACTION POINT

List some things you tell yourself you can't do and rephrase them for a growth rather than fixed mindset.

CHAPTER 24

Understand your behaviour

Have you read *Man's Search for Meaning* by Viktor E. Frankl, an autobiography based on his experiences in various Nazi concentration camps? If you haven't, it's one I recommend. When I'm feeling a bit rubbish, I pick it up for a quick flick through. It's not an obvious choice for a book to turn to when you're needing your soul soothed, but I love it. Viktor Frankl says, "Everything can be taken from a man but one thing, the last of the human freedoms, to choose one's attitude in any given set of circumstances, to choose one's own way."

Now, he was busy choosing his attitude in far harder circumstances than I have ever had to and the freedoms that were taken from him are almost too much to bear thinking about. I certainly don't compare my experience to his, but I can deeply value his thoughts on the subject of choosing one's own way.

In deciding to choose my alcohol-free life experiment, I took a long, hard look at the way my drinking was leading me to behave.

My default behaviour was something like this:

1. I'd drink more than was good for me.

2. I'd think to myself, *Oops, I shouldn't have done that.* (This thought could have popped up after the first sip or when I was six drinks deep.)
3. I'd then feel anxiety or unworthiness and tiredness.

At this low point, I'd have been disappointed with myself, and the behaviour associated with that would have been grumpy, snappy and demotivated. Alcohol wasn't 'making' me behave in a grumpy, snappy or demotivated way. It was a longer journey to get there, involving thoughts and feelings BEFORE the behaviour.

For a quick reality check here, alcohol didn't always result in a negative set of behaviours for me. Sometimes it made me feel sociable and fun. I would, of course, now point out that I always was sociable and fun. It's the atmosphere and the friendship group that makes all the fun possible. I have moments that I look back on and regret. I get these little flashes into my past that bolt out of nowhere every now and again. The idiotic thing I said to a friend of a friend – no harm was meant by it but much offence was caused – a ridiculous conversation with a long-suffering barman, very fancy shoes left in the back of a taxi, an early exit from a beautiful dinner with best friends, too many public toilet puking incidences to mention, and oh so much more. God, this would be a long chapter if I listed thirty years' worth of drinking regrets, but the thing I've come to recognise now – and is the reason that I go back to rethink some of these incidences – is they are so far misaligned with who I want to be now. I really know who I am now. I love going out with my friends and having a fun evening, but I enjoy the simplicity of driving or walking, not booking a taxi. I love laughing at old stories and new jokes. I enjoy going to fun places and remembering it all the next day. I am so happy to always wake up hangover free. I proudly own this behaviour. This is me. This is who I am, who I always could have been bold enough to be, but I wasn't. We all have the right to change our minds over time. Indeed, what is the point of having a mind if not to change and grow?

I used to behave how I did around alcohol because I was insecure and worried about what others would think of me. I used to use alcohol to relax, de-stress and to have fun because I thought it's what everyone did.

Well, newsflash, they don't.

I'm not proud of my past drinking behaviours, but I am pleased with how I behave around alcohol now. I'm not evangelical about a sober life because I very much believe in the mantra 'you do you and I'll do me'. However, I do believe that it's a good thing to let people know that if alcohol is no longer delivering what they thought it would, or is taking more than it should, we can point out a more joyful way of being, leading to behaviours that feel more aligned to you and who you want to be.

ACTION POINT

I invite you to list some new behaviours around alcohol you'd like to move towards.

CHAPTER 25

Cognitive dissonance

Cognitive dissonance is the emotional discomfort we feel when we hold two conflicting beliefs, values or attitudes.

My feelings of emotional discomfort were strong in the early days of my alcohol-free experiment. I wanted to complete my experiment, but I also still believed alcohol helped me to relax and have fun.

The inconsistency between what people believe and how they behave motivates them to engage in actions that will help lessen any feelings of discomfort. People attempt to relieve this tension in different ways, such as by rejecting, explaining away or avoiding new information.

Take these conflicting ideas that you have and examine both sides carefully. See the truth that you really want and discredit the side that isn't supporting you to move towards the life you truly want to be living.

I used to believe that alcohol brought me some benefits AND I also cared about nutrition AND I understood alcohol flavoured with loads of sugar and additives to make it taste nicer was addictive and poisonous AND I knew I hated hangovers and my behaviours when I drank… What inner conflict I had. How glad I am to be free of that now!

ACTION POINT

Can you identify some of your conflicting thoughts around alcohol consumption?

Chapter 26

Limiting beliefs and the lies we tell ourselves

Here is that old favourite Henry T Ford quote: "Whether you think you can, or think you can't – you're right."

We need to start looking at our beliefs around alcohol and decide whether they're helpful to us in achieving the success or the goal we want.

Here are some ideas to start with:

- Old belief: It's not possible to be sober and exciting.
- New belief: It's easier to be more content when I'm sober.

- Old belief: I'm not likeable without alcohol.
- New belief: My sobriety makes me more authentic and present with my friends and family.

- Old belief: Alcohol helps me relax.
- New belief: Sobriety gives me so much more energy in the mornings.

- Old belief: Staying sober is hard.
- New belief: I have all the tools I need to create a brilliant sober life.

- Old belief: Red wine is good for you.
- New belief: Grape juice contains the same benefits as red wine without the toxins.

- Old belief: I need to hit rock bottom before I stop drinking.
- New belief: It's always better to stop a destructive habit while it's still in your control.

- Old belief: Drinking reduces stress.
- New belief: Walking, relaxing on the sofa, yoga, reading, having a bath, phoning a friend all relieve stress.

ACTION POINT

Grab a pen and piece of paper/notebook. Make two columns and go for it… old beliefs on one side of the page, new beliefs on the other!

CHAPTER 27

What will other people think?

When I first decided to embark on my alcohol-free experiment, there were a lot of thoughts running through my head. I became a bit paralysed and unable to move forward for a while because my thoughts were running my feelings and emotions, which were keeping me in that stuck place.

One of the reasons I was so stuck was because I became overly worried about what other people would think about my choice to stop drinking. I found all sorts of ways to soften the blow for friends and family and to change their way of thinking about my choice. I'd say, "Oh, I'm just not drinking today," or, "I'm taking a break for a month," to illustrate that I didn't have a problem with alcohol, and to stop them trying to encourage me to drink. But, of course, trying to make someone think a certain way is impossible, people are going to think what they're going to think and there's only so much you can do to influence that and absolutely nothing you can do to control it. So maybe just stop trying.

While we're here talking about what other people are thinking, you do know that's none of your business, don't you? I say this with love and kindness. What you think of other people is your own private world and the same is true the other way round.

It's really easy to get hung up on explaining ourselves; from why we've made the alcohol-free or sober choice we have, to explaining our drink of choice on a night out. Perhaps you've got a night out planned, either with people you know well or with acquaintances. These might be people who have seen you in your drinking heyday, or people to whom you are a drinking clean slate. We might think, *Oh, what will I say if someone asks what I'm drinking? What if they ask me why I'm not drinking? What if the waiter says there's no alcohol-free beer?"*

Well, I'm going to tell you this. If someone asks what you're drinking, you tell the truth. Tonic water, lime and soda, ginger beer, whatever. If someone asks why you're not drinking, you smile sweetly and either tell the truth, "I'm taking a break at the moment … I feel better not drinking … I don't feel like it tonight," or you tell a white lie if you have to: "I'm on antibiotics … I'm training for a marathon … I'm pregnant." With those last two, be careful, you may need to actually run a marathon or produce a baby at some point. The point is, we think people are interested and we think they care but I'm here to tell you, they really don't. Once they've had one or two drinks themselves, they won't even notice who else is or isn't drinking around them. People occasionally question it when they feel defensive about their own drinking habits, but again, that's on them and not on you. Who cares what other people think, really?

Which are the other areas of your life where you think, *Oh, I wonder what x-y-z friends or colleagues will make of my choice to be… I don't know… vegetarian, getting a dog or painting your sitting room dark green?* Never. You'd just never feel the need to explain or justify your choice, would you?

What will other people think of my choice? The answer is, we have no way of knowing unless we ask them, so you can either ask them or you can be left guessing. But how about this? Don't ask them. And don't guess either. It doesn't matter what anyone else thinks.

It really, really matters what *you* think. And what do you think? I hope it's something along the lines of, *I'm choosing not to drink because I don't want to or need to, I think better, I feel better, and I behave like a more authentic version of myself without it.*

That, my friend, is a good feeling.

ACTION POINT

The *circles of control* tool on the next page helps me to be very clear about what I can control and what I can't and therefore gives me the opportunity to 'let some of it go.'

Circles of control

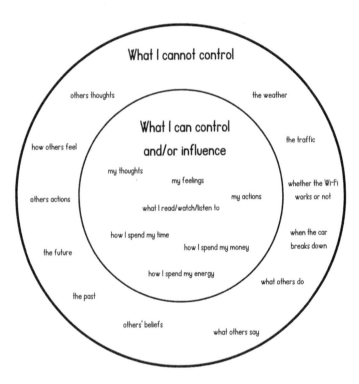

CHAPTER 28

The 'should' siren

Over recent years, I've become more and more aware of my internal dialogue. I think I first really started to listen to myself at the start of my drink less journey. I realised I was having an internal conversation with myself that sounded a bit like this: *I'm not going to drink during the week this week. I probably deserve just one glass of wine. Oh, that would be breaking my own rule. Why can't I ever stick to what I promised myself?* On and on the chat went. The very first step on the way to change was becoming aware of this dialogue. It was bringing attention to the ongoing internal chat and, once there was awareness, I was able to question it. Hmm, how kind and compassionate is that voice in my head? Would I speak to a friend like that? Is that voice even correct? Once I had a first level of awareness, I was able to notice some patterns and words that kept popping up over and over again.

'Should' and 'shouldn't' featured very regularly. *I shouldn't be drinking this. I should be getting up early tomorrow. I shouldn't go out on a Friday and a Saturday night. I should spend some more time playing with my kids.* Relentless, relentless, relentless.

Here is one of the things I find tricky with the 'should' and 'shouldn't' words: whenever I use them, I know there is an implied negativity.

For example, I *should* start meditation and yet I don't.

I *shouldn't* be eating this and yet I am.

I *should* get that job done but I don't know where to start.

I *shouldn't* feel like this but I do.

There's a follow on to this. Because I'm not doing the thing or being the person I think I should be, it means I'm not being the best version of myself. Perhaps I'm lazy. Perhaps I'm not motivated enough. Perhaps I'm not even functioning like a proper human being.

So, to try and help, I've identified the 'should siren'. Whenever I hear the 's' word in my head, I pause to question it and ask myself if it's true.

Here are a couple of reframes:

"I should get up and do that fitness class this morning" changes to "I want to get up and do that class." Here's the thing, I don't necessarily want to get up and do that class, but I do want the benefits of feeling strong and feeling accomplished, knowing I'm looking after myself physically. I focus on how the activity fits with my values.

"I should record my podcast this morning" changes to "I get to record my podcast this morning. I do this every week. I consistently provide this content for an ever-growing audience and I love it."

"I shouldn't feel like this" becomes "I'm noticing how I feel right now. I'm a bit uncomfortable. I'm not sure if

I want to journal about it, talk about it or ignore it at the moment. It's confusing, and I'm wondering why it's like this, and perhaps I will feel a bit better later."

Shall we try to become a bit more conscious of the words should and shouldn't? Let's allow ourselves time, practice and patience to do so. Let's work on a more helpful internal dialogue and hope it leads to a kinder relationship with ourselves. Having the words 'should siren' in my mind is really helpful. I hope it helps you too.

ACTION POINT

Can you write down something you 'should' or 'shouldn't' do this week and reframe it?

CHAPTER 29

How far we've come

I keep two London travel cards. One is dated June 2017 and one is dated June 2022. Almost exactly five years apart. Why do I keep a travel card from five years ago? That day I travelled to London and had a lovely day and then a normal night out. I used to work in the West End, I had the job of my dreams, worked with lovely people and was living my best life – 'working hard; playing hard' as the saying goes. Since I stopped working in London, I regularly visit for an exhibition or theatre trip and drinks or dinner with friends. Well, the June 2017 visit was similar to any other around that time in my life. I had a lovely day out and then met two friends for cocktails followed by dinner. We were trying to remember specifics of the date recently – who else was with us, which bar we went to, where we went to eat, whether we had any pictures on our phones, but no, no recollection. What I can tell you for sure was that I'd had too much to drink before dinner, I carried on drinking wine with dinner, I may well have thrown up partway through the evening and one of my friends would have walked me back to the station and put me on the last train home. He'd have called me a station before my home station to wake me up or remind me to get off and then he'd have called me again to make sure I got home OK (I could pass judgement on myself here – but I won't – I'll just say what an amazing friend I have)! Anyhow, the next day I had a hangover. Well, no surprise there. And it was pretty hideous, probably about an eight-and-a-half out of ten on the hangover scale, or towards one of the inner circles of hell in *Dante's Inferno*.

I remember I had a standout thought on that day in 2017 – something's got to change. I didn't say my usual 'never again' because I'd already said that eleven-billionty times before and I'd never meant it. But this time, *Something's got to change* was a thought and a feeling accompanied by a deep knowing that it was true.

I'm here to tell you that, unfortunately, I carried on drinking and having nights out like that for another eighteen months before I was able to spend a year getting a grip on what that change might look like. By the time we went out in summer 2019, I was able to drink without getting plastered, I was able to have a day and night out in London, have one glass of wine, a lovely dinner, get the train home safely and feel OK the next day. By winter 2019, I had stopped drinking. In the past five years, I'd spent two and a half years preparing to stop drinking and two and a half years without a drink. That is why I keep those two travel cards – to remind myself how hard I've worked and how far I've come.

When we were out in London a few weeks ago, we hung out at a gallery, went for a lovely walk, had dinner and drinks (all alcohol-free) in a brilliant little restaurant we found by accident. We talked a lot about what changes the last five years has brought for us both. When I think about the next five years, I get a bit emotional because I had no idea five years ago that I'd be where I am now, and I had no idea how much better I'd be feeling. It hasn't all been OK. There have been two diagnoses of lifelong critical conditions in my immediate family, deaths and other losses, my own two surgeries and radiotherapy, but, on balance, it's been better. These most recent years have been better. I've felt I've really lived better.

Oh, *Drink Less; Live Better* – there's a good idea.

ACTION POINT

How far have you come already? Can you note down any changes you've made in recent days, weeks or months?

CHAPTER 30

Overcoming overwhelm

Overwhelm can be an everyday underlying feeling or one that hits us at particular times of the year. One thing that has served me really well over the last few years is to only say yes to things if it feels like a *hell yes*. "Yes, I really want to do that. Yes, I want to come with you. Yes, I want to be there." If those are my feelings, then I'm going to go and I'm going to have a nice time. If my feelings are a little bit lukewarm about an invitation, I am so much more likely to turn it down – kindly and politely – now. I value much more time by myself and choosing carefully what I want to do with it is important to me. What are you already committed to? What did you say yes to that now perhaps you're not feeling 100% on? Can you potentially get out of it? If you can't, can you go to it for a shorter time if possible? Enjoy it while you're there but then look forward to leaving? Did you say yes to invitations when you were drinking and, actually, you're not that person any more? So, perhaps you said yes to an invitation like a day at the races and, at the time it was booked, you were looking forward to the amazing day out. Now things are different for you, you're no longer that drinking person. Is it easier to duck out entirely? Or is it

OK to go to that day at the races and enjoy it without a drink? Can you get comfortable with turning up as you are? Can you say, "Yes, I am this person enjoying this day out, and actually, I'm just not drinking, the drinking part is a tiny, tiny bit of who I was and now that's no longer a part of who I am and it also won't be in the future."

Have you got an invitation to a wedding? Weddings are often long, long days. There's the ceremony, a lovely, beautiful celebration of love, where all the focus is on the bride and groom, enjoying the whole service, then outside hopefully to throw the confetti, chat, smile, enjoy some fabulous photos. And then often there's a bit of random standing around before you move towards the next bit of the day. How can you navigate the bit after? Maybe you're really looking forward to chatting to the friends that you're going with or the family that are going to be there. Perhaps you get to the reception and, as you arrive, there's a drinks tray on the way in with all of the glasses of fizz on it. I went to a wedding recently, and as I walked into the reception with my husband, he picked up a glass of fizz and there were two or three waiters there holding the trays and I said to one of them, "Is there an alcohol-free option on the tray?" And they said, "Oh, no, there was some elderflower, hang on a minute, no, I think the kids have drunk it all. Why don't you go to the bar and ask if there's anything there."

I walked through empty handed and, you know what, I don't mind about that kind of thing, but some people get some real security from having a drink in their hand and there could have been loads of drivers who were at that wedding, there may have potentially been people who were pregnant or on medication or like me just chose not to be drinking. And then the onus is on us to go and walk to the bar, which is fine, like I say, I don't mind. I got to the bar and yeah, all of the elderflower had gone and that was fine. I hope they enjoyed it. The option for me was water because this happened to be a fancy bar that was not serving any fizzy drinks or the like. Getting over hurdles like that, for some people, feels like a big deal and for others will feel like a small deal, but they are just part of navigating a whole bigger day.

Are you comfortable standing around chatting at a wedding, potentially with people you don't know? If you need to escape for a while, do it. Go out to your car in the car park, maybe listen to a short podcast (wouldn't it be handy if there was a – oh, I don't know – five or ten-minute podcast that you could just reset and listen to? Oh! There is?! See the *Drink Less; Live Better* podcast!). Maybe go for a walk around the garden. If you're staying at the venue, slip up to your room for a bit of time alone or a quick nap. In my drinking days, I thought I was an extrovert, and I would have loved every moment of being around other people at a wedding. I'd have enjoyed chatting to new people and making new friends. I always left a wedding with several new best friends for life (!). Now I don't drink, I realise that I'm much more introvert. I'm really happy in my own company and, on a long day like a wedding, I need some strategies to survive – it's a great tactic to just take a few breaks.

After the chatting/photos bit, there's all the eating and more drinking, then there might be a bit before the evening bit and then the bit with either the band or the disco. So many moving parts of the day. Just take little breaks whenever you need to. Make sure you tell somebody else that you're OK and that you're happy, that you don't mind at all about not drinking and being around people who are drinking (if that's true). If you're not feeling 100%, make sure you do the right things for you.

Lots of this advice applies if you're at a festival, or any other kind of big party. Make sure you let somebody know that you are OK sitting and watching what's going on if you're not wanting to be involved in everything. I had a really awkward experience recently. I was at a festival and someone came up to me and said, "Oh, you're not dancing at the moment, Sarah, what's going on? You're normally first on the dance floor and we can't get you off." Then she paused and she looked at me and she said, "Oh God. Yes. I've just remembered you don't drink any more." I watched her complete the mental calculations in her head… *Sarah would normally be wild and completely mad on the dance floor, plus, oh yes, she doesn't drink any more, equals, of course, she's going to be sitting down and being boring.* As I saw all of that flit across her face, I felt upset because I've been to this particular festival twice before totally sober, and she has seen me on the dance floor having fun, but hadn't noticed it before. And in that moment, I did feel a little bit wobbly. Not about my decision to be sober or alcohol-free, but about the way that other people view me. Later on that evening, I was on the dance floor. Hopefully that made her feel better but, of course, what she feels or thinks about me is none of my business. I also recognise I was making up my own story about what was going on in her head – I know I'm not a mind reader and never will be.

Go home! Go home when you're ready. No one else will notice once they've had several drinks themselves. Go home. Either your actual home or your hotel room, your tent, wherever… from a wedding, a party, a festival. Don't worry about anyone else – do what is right for you in the moment.

This summer, if you're going on holiday, make sure it's about your health and well-being this year. Too often we come home from our summer holidays and say that we need a break. We need a rest, we need a holiday to get over our holiday. Wouldn't it be amazing if we came back from our holidays well rested, well hydrated, feeling like we'd had fabulous family time and we're ready to get on with the next bit of our lives?

ACTION POINT

Think about upcoming events and note down how you can plan in extra time, space or contingencies if they don't have great options for alcohol-free drinks.

CHAPTER 31

You're not broken

What's going on for you right now? Are you making some baby steps towards the sober lifestyle you know is within your reach? Are you committed to and loving your alcohol-free life? Are you in the process of learning, practising and perfecting the tools that are going to move you in the right direction soon? Whether you are sober one day, one week, one month, one year or more, congratulations, you are here doing something amazing – you are aware and conscious that you want something different for yourself. That's good news. Great news.

Are you feeling positive, motivated and joyful? Or are you feeling a little bit broken by it all? Well, I'm here to tell you, you're not broken, you absolutely are not. Alcohol may well have brought challenges but that is because alcohol is an addictive substance and not because you are in any way failing.

You might feel exhausted by the merry-go-round of 'I'm going to stop drinking' swiftly followed by 'just one won't hurt', or you might feel frustrated that other people can choose to stop and, you know, just stop, or you might feel angry because this isn't fair.

I hear you... exhausted, frustrated and angry – they are all valid feelings as part of the process, but I'll say it again, you are not broken. You may feel a bit battered and bruised, a bit like you're stuck in *Groundhog Day* or like no one else understands the work that you are doing to break free from the cycle that you've been in. It is important work, though.

What needs breaking is the cycle, not you.

You? You are resourceful. You have brought awareness to something and some feelings you no longer want in your life, and you are moving in the right direction. If you don't feel strong enough now, don't worry, you will find the strength. Keep following positive people who inspire you. Listen to the podcasts, read the books, do the work. You are going to rise. You're going to feel all the feelings and emotions on the way, and you are going to come out the other side. And when you do, you will see then, if you cannot see it now, that you weren't broken, you never were. You were just gathering your strength to be able to move on to the next most precious part of your life.

If you cannot see it for yourself now, know that others can.

ACTION POINT

Repeat after me: I am resourceful, I am resourceful, I am resourceful.

Chapter 32

Hold it lightly

Hold a thought, a feeling, a response, action or behaviour lightly. It can be whatever you'd like it to be. I'm holding something lightly at the moment. I'm holding it in my heart and in my head and thinking about it, feeling around it, but letting it drift away and come back again when it's ready each time. I'm not clinging desperately on to it; I've released my grip. I realised I was almost holding my breath and trying to wrestle my way around it, but I've paused on that way of being, I want to give it the energy it deserves, and that energy is peaceful contemplation, not frantic panic.

The difference between clutching tightly and holding lightly feels like the space between where I might squeeze the life out of something versus the opportunity to gently nurture, grow and develop something into its most beautiful way of being.

Holding tightly feels fearful and doubtful. Holding lightly feels expansive and optimistic.

What are you clinging desperately to right now?

Can you imagine putting the thought or feeling or whatever it is into your hands in front of you?

Go on, actually imagine it.

Now do it.

Now, stretch your hands out and hold them out in front of you.

Really stretch them away.

Then slowly bring them back into you and let them rest in a place that feels good.

Look at that empty space in your hands.

Soften your gaze. Just gently glance. See an image held in your open palms just resting there.

Imagine that the image is weightless, and it could fly away at any moment, but it doesn't. It safely rests right there in front of you. You can move your hands towards you if you like. You could bring the image close to your stomach or your heart.

Or you could just softly watch it unfold right where it is. Let some time pass by you and your vision.

Your grip is loose, but your heart feels full.

Know that by holding it lightly, you're giving it space. You're taking away the desire to control it. Treat it kindly, with reverence, contemplate it and then take aligned action.

But just don't squeeze the life out of it. OK?

ACTION POINT

This whole chapter is an action, so follow this process through as often as you need/want to.

CHAPTER 33

Contrast

Living a life at opposite ends of the spectrum and everywhere in between brings me joy and balance. I love London. It's a beautiful city. I live about an hour away and regularly go in for a day. I love the bustle. I love the busy. I love the buildings. I love the friends that I hang out with when I'm in London. I also love wide open spaces, the sea, open fields and woodlands. I also live just over an hour away from the sea. I love the silence of a deserted beach. I love pebbles (not sand – if you're interested) under foot. I love the sound of waves hitting the shore. I love distant horizons.

The contrast between city and sea. There's a time for city busy and a time for big blue nature. It's the difference between fast and slow. It's two opposites but also both big and expansive, full of potential. It's also the difference between spending time with people who I love and spending time in solitude. I never feel lonely when I am alone. I love my own company for chunks of time. It also feels like the difference between superficial quick conversations and deep, deep time in thought. It's also the difference between other people's opinions and my opinions. It's dark to light.

There are contrasts of avoiding what's going on versus facing reality and gently, lovingly accepting it. The difference between desperately, desperately wanting something and actually choosing it. The difference between feeling suspicious and anxious versus trusting. And also, the difference between something feeling grim and heavy versus lighthearted. There's so much contrast, so many differences. I'm comfortable now that apparently conflicting ideas/concepts can be true at the same time.

ACTION POINT

Where are the contrasts in your life at the moment? Do they feel OK to you

CHAPTER 34

If not now, when?

I can be masterful at putting something off. And I mean masterful. I can have a variety of tasks outstanding, some of them are urgent and important, some urgent, some are important. Some are neither urgent nor important but do need my attention soonish. Some should be delegated and should never have snuck onto that list in the first place; and just as soon as I'm bold enough, I'm going to get rid of them. Not now, though, later. I've got to delete them later because first I need to overthink them, I need to ask other people's opinions, I need to take them off the list, then put them back on. I also need to see who else has those things on their list and ask them how they took them off or ask why they left them on. I know that, deep down, I want to delete those tasks, but I am afraid to, I don't know what will happen if I do.

Can you see where I'm going with this? Let's pop drinking into the 'deleting a task' box. If I'm going to consider a break from booze, a drink less experiment or a period of sobriety, I need to ask my friends what they think of my choice. I need to decide then change my mind. I need to know who else isn't drinking and ask them why.

Maybe I know, deep down, I'd really benefit from a break from drinking, but it feels enormous and putting it off is preferable to taking action right now. Is the pain of changing worse or better than the pain of staying the same? If the pain of change would be better embraced... then when? When is the right time?

I'm going to tell you straight up that *now* is the answer. Now will always be my answer. As soon as you finished your drinking or when you are done with the hangovers, the low-level brain fog, the rubbish nutritional and exercise choices you are making: you are done.

If not now, then when? I've been honest, I took a long time to get finished with drinking. I had excuses to make before I could get to the start line.

If not now, when? Is it after that wedding? The fortieth or fiftieth birthday party? The festival? Yeah, yeah, I know, I know. We think we have to drink at all of these events. Guess what, dear friend? We don't. We absolutely do not.

Tell me, what makes you think that you should? Is it because it's what you've always done? Is it because it's what everybody else is doing? Is it because you're worried about what everyone else will say?

I'm here to tell you: it's OK. Yes, those are valid thoughts. They'll be valid today and tomorrow, next week, next month and after the wedding, the birthday and the festival. You will always tell me a reason why it cannot be now and I'll ask you again: if not now, when?

Choose now because now is ideal. Even if you choose now and choose it until the wedding, the party, the festival, you will have lined up a whole load of days of learning how it is to lead a drink less or sober lifestyle and, maybe, just maybe, at that point, you won't feel like drinking at that event anyway. So, it's no longer a problem.

If not now, when? You already know Mondays aren't good for new habits. You know the first of January isn't brilliant for a year-long resolution. So what's making you think that a future point is going to be the Holy Grail?

Go on. I dare you. Start now.

ACTION POINT

If not now, when?

Write that date down! Take the first action.

PART 3

ACTION

"Action is the foundational key to success."
Pablo Picasso

CHAPTER 35

OK, go!

You are already 'in action', you're reading this book!

It's a new season of your life, maybe a new month, a new notebook, a blank page, an opportunity to draw a line underneath something and crack on with building the next exciting bit. You're allowed to start anew and be a beginner when you are trying on a new lifestyle, learning new habits and/or experimenting.

Sometimes a big deal is made about starting points. There's a lot of talk about making a change and picking a future date to dig in and get started, and that's truly great if that works for you. Ultimately, picking a future date for changes is a bit of an anti-climax for me. NOW, today, positive forward action and momentum works best of all. You don't have to wait to change. Now is good.

My experience of choosing a date to make the significant life change of being alcohol-free for one year went a bit unexpectedly as I outlined in Chapter 2. I had begun to cut my drinking down significantly, I was considering my next step and had got my head around the idea of a year without alcohol, but I was waiting until the end of December to begin. In my mind, a year has a very clear start and finish

– 1st of January to 31st of December – right? All new things must start on the 1st of January – it's a rule of life, isn't it? It's called a New Year resolution for a reason. Now, depending on what source you want to believe, as many as 80% of New Year resolutions come to a sticky end in the month of January, so your chances of success aren't looking good before you've even begun. During 2019, I had the realisation that there was no point in waiting for the right moment to start my alcohol-free experiment. The only time I would be ready was NOW. If I hung on, there would be a wedding, a birthday, a Friday night or… coming right up was Christmas, New Year and whatever other reason I came up with!

I concluded that if I started now then I could get all the slightly tricky Christmas events under my belt and then start January feeling a bit smug and as if all the hard events had already been tackled alcohol-free.

For me, new beginnings and new habits happen when they feel good. My alcohol-free life experiment continues and now allows me the opportunity to add other great things into my life that I didn't quite have the time or inclination for before.

If there's a new beginning wanting to get out, allow it, listen to your intuition, give yourself space, be bold. If it's something you think other people may have an opinion about, just remember: what other people think of us or our ideas is always none of our business.

You pick your lane and stay in it.

If you need help or support to be successful with your new beginning, then look for other people who have already got some of what you want. You'll find them, your people are out there doing the same thing as you in their own way – follow and/or engage with them.

Choosing a new habit can be difficult to start with and, with an alcohol habit, the most difficult bit can be days one to fourteen. Unfortunately, many people spend a lot of time repeating days one to fourteen. I did. In fact, I probably spent about two and a half years thinking I was going to stop drinking, stopping for a bit, starting again and repeat, repeat, repeat!

I never really got to know how good it felt at weeks three or four and beyond because I was trapped in a bit of a cycle I couldn't break. I experienced bits of elation (*yay, one week without a drink – aren't I fabulous?*) to lots of doom (*damn it – failed again*) to celebration (*yes, I can do this*) to huge withdrawal headache (*that hurts – I'll have a drink to take the edge off*) to OK, *I'll try again today* before it really started to stick.

When I finally set the goal I wanted to achieve, questioned EVERYTHING around my drinking habits and the cultural conditioning I'd been exposed to, developed tools to help my cravings and triggers, got clear on my values, chose alternative socialising habits and STOPPED tripping myself up, it all fell into place.

ACTION POINT

Are you what you repeatedly do? What new habits are you forming?

CHAPTER 36

A quick tip for the early days

Have you ever heard the acronym HALT?

Apart from the word itself meaning 'stop', the acronym stands for **H**ungry, **A**ngry, **L**onely or **T**ired and can be used as a mindset tool in a wide variety of situations, not least those involving eating and drinking. The model was originally developed to help people in recovery see when they might be vulnerable to returning to old habits.

How do you feel right now? Can you stop for a moment and really recognise where you are emotionally? Do you feel great? OK? Not so good?

If you aren't feeling your greatest, taking a moment to HALT is one of the best things you can do for your overall mental and physical health. Here is how I used this tool when I was first alcohol-free.

The moments in my life when I was most likely to reach for a drink at home was sometime after 6pm when the day felt like it was about to change gear out of work mode and into either cooking time, family time, relaxation time or perhaps socialising.

HALT

Hunger

At 5pm, when I was standing in the kitchen thinking about cooking, it was all too easy to reach for something to eat quickly (which was generally unhealthy), but what I really needed at that time was a large glass of water. I made a conscious effort to switch my afternoon snacking habit to make sure I always had a good snack and large glass of water at about 4pm in the afternoon instead of waiting until I was ravenous and therefore more likely to want to press the self-destruct button and pour myself a glass of wine.

I often mistook hunger for thirst and used wine as a thirst quencher. Recognising I was allowing myself to feel so depleted resulted in a relatively easy fix.

Anger

For me, it was easier to describe my anger as feeling generally unwanted emotions – I wasn't always able to think rationally when in a certain mindset. I had to learn to recognise the emotions and find ways to process them.

Alcohol might temporarily numb the feeling of anger, but it certainly won't relieve the cause of the anger.

Loneliness

Most of us experience loneliness at times in our lives. Even when people surround us in a busy family, we may not be actively interacting with them, and the feeling of isolation can feel even more surprising. What's more, with all our modern technology, many of us are plugged in electronically but not connected emotionally.

I used to stand gazing into the fridge wondering what I was looking for and it took me a long time to realise that over the years I'd taken to phoning my friends less. Before we had kids, we used to speak on the phone regularly, and somehow life had got in the way of that lovely practice and had been replaced by text messages or other quick typed notes. I've reintroduced the practice of phone calls with friends and feel much more connected and less lonely.

A glass of wine won't ever fix lonely!

Tiredness... or exhaustion... or overwhelm

I used to get to 5pm and think that it was now time to turn off. I didn't have a strategy that allowed me to happily change pace and a glass of wine or G and T in my hand felt like a little 'pick me up' or treat to see me through a task that didn't fill me with all the joy in the world, i.e. cooking dinner. I looked for new ways to treat myself at this time. A ten-minute walk around the block to reinvigorate myself, a five-minute guided meditation to calm myself, a few yoga stretches to remove tension from my body, a phone call to a friend, listening to a podcast – these were all strategies that worked brilliantly. I kept a list of ideas in the back of my diary so I didn't have to think of them – I could just open the page and pick something. When you are already tired, it's difficult to come up with new strategies to cope. Be prepared.

A drink never did help me feel less tired, it just helped to mask the feeling of overwhelm. How can you start to remove the overwhelm from your life, so you don't arrive at 5pm feeling like a drink is the only option?

Some of the emotions mentioned here felt horrible when I first started to identify them in myself. I didn't want to admit that I was lonely – I've got a loving family living in the same house as me and I've got fabulous friends who are round the corner or on the end of the line.

I have a sticky note with HALT written on it inside the cupboard where I used to keep my gin. The note is still there and the gin has been replaced with alcohol-free gin, fancy tonics and other delicious drinks. I leave the note there as a little celebration for myself that the tool of alcohol is no longer needed to cope with my emotions.

Designing a life you don't need alcohol to escape from is part of the key to sober success, and making sure I had a range of mind, body and soul nourishing tools to use to make that life a reality is something that has brought me joy and peace of mind.

ACTION POINT

Grab those sticky notes, write HALT on them and stick them in the places you need reminders.

Think: Eat/hydrate, process emotions, connect and rest

CHAPTER 37

Eat well and hydrate

When I used to drink, I used to snack at the same time. I LOVED snacking. Salted, roasted nuts – yes please. Crisps/ chips – yes please. Japanese crackers – yes please. Olives – yes please. Cheese straws – yes please… you get the picture!

I ate and drank to excess most evenings and I had NO CLUE that one habit was fuelling the other. I thought I snacked because dinner wasn't ready yet and I was going to eat my own arm if someone didn't feed me now. I was often hungry and grumpy and not the very best version of me at the same time of day that my kids were fractious!

When I stopped drinking and got into the habit of having a proper, nutritious snack mid-afternoon (and a large glass of water), my early evening snacking habit disappeared completely.

However, the thing that took me by surprise was the sugar cravings. I never used to go mad for chocolate but, for a few months after I stopped drinking, I really craved sugar in that way and I just 'went with it' for a while. I was so happy not to be drinking.

After a couple of months, I was able to leave the chocolate aside and get on without too many cravings. I was conscious of what was happening in my body, and I want you to be too. Go with the food you need at the time you need it.

Also... hangover eating! Can I tell you this... since I stopped drinking, I haven't HAD to eat cake for breakfast once. I also have not had to eat fried egg and chips or have a fizzy drink for breakfast AND... I also no longer drink three coffees before I can leave the house!

All WINS in a big way, I think you'll agree!

Do you know how much water you should drink in a day? Part of the reason I used to hit my first glass of wine in the evening was because I was thirsty. I didn't realise it at the time, but I wasn't drinking enough fluid during the day.

When I had stopped drinking and started to investigate how much water I should drink, I was really put off by all the differing advice.

Instead, see the action point with the best calculation by a nutritionist friend of mine to find out how much water your body needs to function efficiently.

I bought a lovely water bottle that holds exactly half of what I need in a day. I fill and drink it once in the morning and the same in the afternoon.

No more thirsty wine craving!

ACTION POINT

Weigh yourself in kilograms.

Then multiply the number of kilos you weigh by 0.033.

This will give you the amount you need to drink in litres.

For example, if you weighed 65kg:

65 x 0.033 =2.1

Your water intake would need to be 2.1 litres.

SIMPLE!

CHAPTER 38

Finding joy in an alcohol-free world

I wasn't not living a jolly life – excuse the double negative but it's true. Everything was OK. Well, better than OK, actually, everything was going well. I've mentioned it before… a lovely husband, gorgeous kids, nice house, dog, friends, extended family, job and ALL THE THINGS. Did you read that? I typed it in capitals just to be clear: ALL THE THINGS. All the things make a person happy and fulfilled, don't they?

I was OK but I had an underlying feeling of unease, a niggle, a deep sense that things could be better than they were, but I couldn't put my finger on it.

So, I did what any sane and rational person would do in an already full life – I added more. More to do, more to be, more to remember, more to make time for, more to pay for.

I added yoga because all yogis are enlightened.

I added green smoothies because they make you beautiful.

I added meditation because who is more zen and happier than a Buddhist monk.

I added vitamins because someone told me to (although they didn't mention that they only work if you use them and you don't leave them sitting on your kitchen counter top).

I added running because… well, that's a surefire way to move you further away from your problem physically (!).

And all the problem-solving ideas didn't solve the problem.

I decided I'd do away with alcohol for a year and was sure this would lead to a further sense of dissatisfaction because I was clearly going to spend a year being bored, miserable and lonely.

I had no idea what was to come.

Now, let's be quite clear at this point. When I stopped drinking, the clouds did not immediately part and rain down magical unicorns, rainbows and golden glitter.

No, there wasn't an immediate stratospheric rise to the top of the emotions scale. However, that feeling of unease dissipated, the low-level brain fog, the rumbling anxiety all lifted over time. I hadn't noticed how much I had been entertaining negative thought patterns and voices in my head until I stopped hearing them so much.

I started to feel excited and passionate about my alcohol-free life experiment and I sought out like-minded people who were totally happy about their life choice.

I got into and enjoyed conversations, connections and collaborations.

I spent more time in real life with the people who made me feel good.

I changed my socialising habits to coffees, brunches and dog walks.

I brought colour back into my wardrobe – I stopped wearing grey every day and chose brights instead.

I bought houseplants and didn't kill them.

I moved my body.

I got outside.

I started helping and supporting other people.

Instead of pursuing happiness externally, I began to feel it deeply within me when I wasn't looking for it.

As I got further and further away from my last drink and the anxiety subsided, I found it easier and easier to connect with my feelings of contentment and peace.

Where I had simplified my life a bit and made time for what was really important to me, I found joy in a good book, an hour of sewing or painting, a long bath or an excellent cup of tea.

When the tough stuff is happening around me, I try to see the good bits in the situation. I had four visits to hospital in six days recently, but I chose to focus on the shared drives there and back with my son, the easy access to transport, the lovely hospital we go to, the nice staff we see. I don't ignore the bad stuff – I just don't give it the energy I would've done years ago.

No drama, thank you.

So, there you have it. Joy. For me, it's an inside job, it was taking alcohol away and seeing all the good stuff that was there for the recognising and making.

ACTION POINT

Is there a place in your life you can release a bit of drama or chaos? Note it down if it's useful to come back to.

CHAPTER 39

Cravings

The bad news: Cravings can take up a large amount of head space in the first few weeks of going alcohol-free.

The good news: There are tools we can use to help us through the early days, and we can go back to the same tools over and over again in the future, if we need to.

One thing is for certain – the first stint of going alcohol-free is likely to be the hardest. So, the best thing you can do is start to put some serious distance between now and your last drink so that you don't have to keep on repeating the painful cycle of stopping again and again.

I accept cravings can be tricky to deal with. Distraction is a technique that works well for some people in the early days of their sobriety. Moving environments (going for a walk), getting some support (phoning a sober friend), educating yourself (reading a sobriety memoir or listening to a podcast) can be helpful.

Cravings are physical and psychological experiences. If you look after your body, you can minimise the impact of the cravings – if you eat well, hydrate, exercise and sleep, you'll be less vulnerable.

If you concentrate on your mind and listen to the 'stories' you are saying to yourself about the cravings, you will be able to analyse them and then take alternative actions to pouring a drink.

Some people find they suddenly crave sugary snacks when they first stop drinking. I did too. I decided that I would 'give in' to my newfound sweet tooth temporarily while I got a good stretch of sobriety under my belt. I knew I was best off tackling the alcohol first and the sugar at a later date.

Practising these new skills will bring progress and then, later on, perfection!

Some people refer to the moments where your emotional state is shifted momentarily as a trigger – a trigger might affect your ability to remain present in the moment and it may bring up specific thought patterns or influence your behaviour differently than you would like. If I ever feel myself getting wistful or romanticising the idea of having an alcoholic drink, I have a few sentences in the back of my head I can reach for:

- No one ever regretting NOT drinking the morning after.
- I've made my AF choice tonight and I'm delighted with my decision.
- I am fuelled by the people I'm with and the fun I share with them.
- Alcohol poisons my body and brain and tomorrow morning I'll feel fabulous.
- I choose alcohol-free and joy-filled experiences.

If I'm momentarily struggling, I question the struggle, confirm with myself that I'm not giving in in this moment and then I recommit to it by saying inside my head: *This moment is fleeting.*

I find positive words to reframe the situation when I feel a wobble, I stop and breathe – really breathe – for a moment, I choose delicious food and really enjoy it, I check in with my alcohol-free friends and I stand firm. I might question my decision from time to time, but I always come back to it as the right choice.

ACTION POINT

I use the affirmation: *This moment is fleeting.* Could you use the same sentence or does something else seem more *you?*

CHAPTER 40

What do you drink instead of alcohol?

I knew there was water, and I knew there was juice, and that was fine to start with. One of the issues I'd come to realise over time was that I've never drunk enough water. When I'd got stuck into a glass of wine at the end of the day, it had always been in part as a thirst quencher. Drinking more water during the day was a brilliant starting point, meaning come 5pm I wasn't dehydrated.

The first thing I missed was my Thursday night G and T. Part of what I loved about my G and T was the ritual of getting a nice heavy glass out, cutting a lime, clinking the ice into the glass and then pouring the drink before leaning back on the counter and taking a large gulp. So... I made a really simple switch to a non-alcoholic gin. I get the same feeling of my Thursday ritual but with none of the negative side effects of the alcohol. Perfect.

Have you ever heard of kombucha? I hadn't. It's a fermented, lightly sparkling, flavoured tea drink. There are loads of brands and flavours out there or you can make your own. I started drinking it from time to time as a replacement for white wine.

In a pub, I love a ginger beer, a lime and soda or an alcohol-free lager if they have one. If I'm out with my girlfriends, I'll quite often have a flavoured tonic in a fancy gin glass.

I've found lots of nice, flavoured waters, iced teas, alcohol-free fizzes and I also love making my own alcohol-free mocktails.

I've never felt deprived, which, in a way, I'm quite surprised by.

It's the atmosphere, the company, the fun times I crave – not the alcohol.

ACTION POINT

What are the drinks you are going to choose now? What have you tried and enjoyed before and what do you want to test out?

CHAPTER 41

Who do you tell/share with when you choose to drink less or go alcohol-free?

You don't owe anyone an explanation (and certainly not an apology) for your choice to drink less or not drink at all. You don't need permission. You don't need an opinion.

You don't need anyone to say, "Oh, you're not that bad really," or, "You're no worse than the rest of us," or, "Why don't you just have a couple?"

Some of the conversations you start to have with family, friends or acquaintances will be uncomfortable, but they will also get easier and eventually become a thing of your past.

The first time I said I was going to go alcohol-free for a year was on a video group coaching call in 2019 where we were discussing some new goals we all hoped to be working towards. I loved the people and the facilitator, and it was an uplifting and joyful group to be in. As we went around the group declaring our goals, I said, "I'm not going to say mine out loud, thanks, I'm keeping it in my head."

The conversation moved on and dreams were discussed,

plans were put in place and futures were talked about as possible realities. Towards the end of the session, someone said, "Come on, Sarah, the suspense is killing me, what's your goal and why won't you share it?"

The second part of that question was easy: "If I share it, it will feel real and then I'll have to follow through on it."

The first part – not so easy... I took a deep breath and then said: "I'm going to be alcohol-free in 2020."

Silence.

Tumbleweed.

Well, I'd pretty much just declared myself to be miserable, lonely and boring, hadn't I? What *can* you expect people to say in that situation?

I fluffed around... "I don't drink more than the government guidelines in an average week, I just drink too much wine more often than I'd like to, I sometimes don't feel my best in the mornings..." I also pointed out that I was only drinking the same amount as everyone else I knew, and I was managing to look after my family, do some yoga, go running, take my vitamins, drink my smoothies and, y'know, generally be a fabulous human in many other ways!

Anyway, the group vibe was one of 'good for you, well done and let us know how it goes!' which was reassuring, and now that I'd said it out loud, it wasn't a secret any more, and that felt good.

Saying my goal in a group setting had made it seem more real and that group had been a safe bet for not feeling judged. I'd plucked up the courage to say it because I wanted other people to know and hold me accountable.

In October 2019, I told my husband I wasn't going to drink in 2020. It was no big conversation, there were no questions from him and no justifications from me – just a comfortable acceptance. We've talked about it since and it's no biggy in our lives. He carried on drinking when I stopped, and my experiment has always been about me and not him or us.

The first couple of times I went out after I'd decided to be alcohol-free was to friends' houses and I didn't tell them about my choice as I wasn't yet ready to chat about it. On those nights, I acted as the barmaid and poured everyone else's drinks for them. When I was in the kitchen, I just topped up my glass with tonic water and everyone assumed I was drinking gin and tonic. The next couple of nights out, I made myself the driver, as that's always a valid reason not to drink and no one I know would question that!

When I was ready to chat to friends, I was careful to mention it outside of drinking situations. If we were out for a dog walk, a coffee or at each other's houses for a cuppa, I chose to mention it then – it felt far less confrontational if neither of us had an alcoholic drink in our hand. I always made it casual and never mentioned the year-long time frame I had in mind. I said, "Oh, I'm just choosing not to drink for the time being and I'm feeling so much better for it." No one tried to change my mind and I was able to feel good about the choice I was making for myself.

As time went on, I became more honest about my intention to be alcohol-free for the whole year, and it did then start attracting statements such as, "Oh, but you don't have a problem, you don't need to punish yourself like that, surely you can just have one or two drinks?" None of which was helpful, obviously!

By this stage, I was really starting to feel the physical and emotional benefits of my alcohol-free experiment and these conversations became easier and easier to have. I didn't have a problem with alcohol, it just wasn't offering me any positive benefits. I'm not punishing myself – I'm doing the opposite, I'm treating myself with great love and kindness. I would be fine having just one or two, but I don't want that any more.

At times, I felt slightly uncomfortable because friends would tell me all the reasons why they were fine drinking. It felt too much like an explanation or justification I hadn't asked for and didn't need.

Whether I drink or don't doesn't come up in conversation much now. Once I was joyful and confident in my choice, it just wasn't questioned any more. Where once I had looked for reassurance from others, I now find it with myself.

ACTION POINT

If someone offers you their advice at any point in your decision-making process, please ask yourself these three questions:

1. Is this person happy with the life they are living?

2. Is this person living a life I would be happy with?
3. Does this person really know what my fears and uncertainties are?

If the answer to any of those questions is no, you may be better finding another adviser or cheerleader!

CHAPTER 42

Relationships

Oh, yes. That heady, heady mix – husband, kids, wider family, old friends, new friends. When I thought of all the different people in my life I had or have relationships with, and what part, if any, alcohol played in them, I started to feel a bit overwhelmed. I'd also forgotten to add myself to the list.

I'd spent years and years thinking that alcohol made me a better version of myself. I thought it made me more sociable, more outgoing, more relaxed, less stressed, less lonely, less boring and, of course, much, much funnier. I had no idea that the better version of me was the one who was sober-powered, not alcohol-fuelled. The bits I chose to spend less time remembering are the stories of repeating myself endlessly, falling over, vomiting, unintentionally offending someone, leaving my shoes in the back of the taxi and, of course, worse. I was convinced I had to play the role of 'the life and soul of the party'. I was first on the dance floor and last off, could always be relied upon to have 'one for the road' at the end of the evening and I thought I was happy.

Well, I suppose I was on the surface. I walked around

with a smile on my face. I live in a nice house in a lovely town with my 'almost normal' family and dog. What could my problem possibly be? Well, duh, obviously, it was my relationship with myself. Hindsight is a wonderful thing and, if I could go back and have a quiet word in the ear of a younger me, I'd say, *Stop. Just stop. Be.* I'd have been in no position to listen, to pay attention or even consider the possibility of a problem. But there was a problem. I couldn't just be, I couldn't be still. I couldn't be quiet. I couldn't be relaxed by myself. I was in a constant state of action and this, this was part of what was wrong. I remember one of my lovely friends asking me if I'd ever tried to meditate and I can really clearly remember my answer: "No, I absolutely do not want to be still and listen to the voice in my head. That would be torture." We laughed and she casually mentioned that maybe that was the exact reason why I should try it, and we moved on. Years later, I knew she saw in me what I wasn't willing to see in myself and, of course, she was right. I'm here to advocate meditation for you, too, if it feels good. For too long, the voice in my head had been critical and scathing, the voice that talked to me at 6pm endlessly mentioned a glass of wine as a reward for getting through the day and the voice in the morning questioned why I drank the wine the night before. The voice wanted to know if I was a good enough mum, a loving enough wife, a caring enough employee, a loving enough friend, whether all the roles I was fulfilling in life were going OK.

What I never asked myself was about my relationship with myself, which I now realise is the most important relationship of all. Making the decision to stop drinking alcohol was the greatest gift I ever gave my relationship with myself. It gave me an opportunity to grow in ways I never would have dreamed of, and the very best thing of all is that the voice in my head – which is, of course, me – is altogether kinder, less judgemental and more forgiving. I can honestly say I much prefer myself now.

ACTION POINT

How is your relationship with yourself at the moment – are you moving towards a more gentle way of treating yourself?

CHAPTER 43

What you say really matters – choose carefully!

"I'm never drinking again," was always uttered at low moments in my life; either right at the end of the drinking night out, just before a restless, sweaty sleep, or in any of the twenty-four, forty-eight or seventy-two hours following an evening of too much alcohol. You see, even though I said it and sometimes meant it, I never truly believed it because, once the dreadful hangover had passed and the self-hatred settled down, I knew I would drink again. I knew deep down that when I said, "I'm never drinking again," it was a big fat lie. Sometimes I even said it in jest. The 'never again' messages in a WhatsApp group were shared around as an almost badge of honour. Oh, how we laughed. We also joked that our feeling terrible was down to food poisoning or other hilarious excuses. I couldn't bring myself to say, "I'm never drinking again," and mean it.

Your words really matter when you are looking for a new reality for yourself. If you talk about how you cannot do something or how you hate something, you're going to be unlikely to make it a part of who you want to be.

Here are some phrases to look out for: I can't, I wish, I

won't, I haven't, I'm rubbish at, I'm trying to. I was known to say, "I can't drink just two glasses of wine. I wish I didn't drink like an idiot. I won't ever succeed at this. I hate myself for this behaviour."

Stopping and reconsidering my language – both about myself and to myself – made such a massive difference. What do you think about these starter phrases: I can, I do, I am, I create, I'm good at, I'm so grateful for, I choose.

Almost any of the rubbish stories I was telling myself could be much more helpfully reframed with the use of these ideas. I can be alcohol-free. I know what's good for me. I create fabulous connections and relationships based on deep and meaningful conversations, not slippery dance floors. I'm good at noticing the benefits of an alcohol-free life experiment. I'm so grateful for boldly making this choice. I choose relaxed and happy over anxious and hungover.

Listen carefully to the words and messages you hear about yourself. Have an out loud response, or if you cannot manage that then an internal one. Here's an example of mine: "Oh, Sarah's always leaving her shoes in the back of a taxi," gets the rebuke of, "Not any more, I'm the taxi driver." Choose yourself a new sentence for the new you. Then say it out loud. Write it down. Believe in it. Become it. Dream it as you fall asleep at night. One of mine was, "I choose to be peacefully alcohol-free." I didn't like words like quit, stop or give up, so this choice of words really suited me. When I'm trying to think of some good words, a turn of phrase, a label or title for something, I'm often to be found scribbling the initial idea down and then turning to my online thesaurus to uplevel my words or find some alliteration that sounds or looks comfortable. I have 'sober is my superpower' written on the noticeboard above my desk as a little reminder of what I want to be, do and share with the world. Well, my tiny corner of the world, any way.

ACTION POINT

I *believe* sober is my superpower. I *trust* sober is my superpower. How about you?

Could you choose something to say about yourself you can believe and trust in?

CHAPTER 44

Is connection the opposite of addiction?

Connection. I'd never really thought about it too much when I was drinking. I'd have told you I had a lovely family, friends, colleagues and clients I worked with, but it means something different to me now and I predict it will change again in the future. If you've not watched the TED talk by Johann Hari, 'Everything you think you know about addiction is wrong', I recommend you look it up and enjoy his wisdom.

Almost everyone I know who works in a similar field to me knows and loves the last line of his talk: "The opposite of addiction is not sobriety, the opposite of addiction is connection." I love that thought too, but I tried to keep in mind that it's a line that's easy to say, and in reality harder for some of us to practise. Johann talks about the 'Rat Park' work of Dr Bruce Alexander, who studied the ways rats became addicted to morphine over short periods of time. Rats in cages in isolation could either drink water or water laced with morphine, and they always chose the morphine version, eventually dying from that choice. The rats who lived in Rat Park – a rat utopia with plenty of stimulation

– also had refreshment choices, but they chose water. The Rat Park rats were, of course, altogether happier rats. Johann tells us that individual recovery is OK, if it works well for you, but that we should perhaps be talking more about social recovery, looking to each other for love and support. As I watched his talk, I began to wonder why I hadn't ever looked for a community of like-minded people when I first knew I was going to go alcohol-free for a year. I know that shame played a big part in my choice not to talk about what I was doing. I judged myself harshly. I mean, people who give up drinking are the ones who really *need* to, the ones who have blown their lives up in a skip fire, the ones who were on the receiving end of an intervention, the ones who pour vodka on their cornflakes for breakfast. Aren't they? Wasn't I?

I didn't know then what I know now. I desperately wanted to feel connected. I wanted to know, love and trust someone slightly further ahead on their journey than I was. I wanted people right alongside me. I also wanted people coming up behind who I could help and support too.

I was not into social media before 2019. I came into it very gently at the start of that year, just to use one specific group initially, which happened to be nothing to do with sobriety. I then began to realise there were groups for just about any subject in the world you'd care to think about. I joined a few groups with sober or alcohol-free in the title and found some groups I loved and some not so much. There were enormous groups with thousands and thousands of people and smaller groups with a few hundred. Some groups run by sober powerhouses, and some by people who had set up their group up in the hope of just finding a few friends. Every group has a different feel, depending on who runs the group, who moderates it and the purpose/ethos of the group. Some groups have some very loud, shouty, opinionated people in and some are run with nothing but love and kindness. I suggest that you do your own research and find the groups that suit you. You will find some groups are focused on one pathway to recovery, and others are more celebratory of all pathways. Of course, not every group is hosted on social media. There are many other communities hidden in all the nooks and crannies of the internet. Some groups are free, and some are paid memberships. Some offer amazing accountability and coaching for support, and it is becoming increasingly common to be able to easily meet other lovely sober people in real life – the total joy of real people, not heads on video screens! You'll find lunches out, dog walks, visits to new places, sober parties, raves and festivals. Yes, yes, yes – there's something to suit every extrovert or introvert. Through sober communities and training courses, I've met new friends – not just acquaintances, but people who really know what I'm all about, who see, hear and understand me, and I do the very same for them. These beautiful souls make everything seem OK on a slightly less than good day. In the future, I can only see more connection, more collaboration, more opportunities to make friends, to share, to belong, to be together. Anyway, all this is to say, don't feel alone in your choice to drink less or be alcohol-free.

There are other people out there making the same rockstar decisions you are and they are just waiting for you to find them. It's true, connection is the opposite of addiction.

ACTION POINT

Don't forget to go and watch Johann's Ted Talk!

https://www.ted.com/talks/johann_hari_everything_you_ think_you_know_about_addiction_is_wrong/c

CHAPTER 45

Accountability

If you're pursuing a short-term goal, it's helpful to put in place tools that will help you to get to where you want to be. What have you been doing to move yourself towards your goal up until now? And is it working?

A word from the wise here: if you are using resources that are not leading to the success or outcome you want then stop right now, put down what isn't working, I give you permission.

Here is my example from about a year ago. The activity was 'set alarm for 6am each weekday morning' because I wanted to go out for a run for one hour before I started my day. The result was 'press snooze button repeatedly' for three months until I turned the bloody alarm off. The feeling was failure. Now I've got six months under my belt of a different behaviour. The activity is 'set alarm for 6.15 three mornings per week' to weight train with a trainer and accountability group. The result is 'lowered heart rate, beautiful arms and shoulders (if I do say so myself) and the feeling of success'. I put my success in this area down to two things. Number one: having a goal that, while outside my comfort zone, I suspected I could do. Number two:

knowing someone else was expecting me at that class.

If what you're doing isn't working, try something else. Be accountable, be accountable to a close friend who understands, be accountable to an internet friend who understands, spend your drinking money on a support/sober/recovery coach, either one-to-one or in a group. Go to AA or SMART meetings. Don't get caught up in hiding. Declare your short-term goals and don't retreat when the going gets tough. Use your accountability partner or group to talk through your values and what motivates you, work on your limiting beliefs, your mindset, your thought patterns and behaviour change. Change in a good and powerful way. Let go of the stories that might be holding you back. Take the action. If you don't know what the action is, then get help with that first.

Accountability will help you to commit, you'll be more dedicated to your goal and more motivated to keep moving forward.

Accountability will help you get really clear on the tools and resources you'll need both now and in the future. What are the things you must be, do or share to be successful in your goal?

Accountability helps you be creative. If you hit a roadblock, there's a sounding board to help you find the way through.

Accountability increases your competence. When you know someone else is watching you, you tend to focus better.

Accountability gives you an opportunity to celebrate.

You'll have a cheerleader who will celebrate all the milestones with you.

Commitment, clarity, creativity, competence and celebration. These are just some of the things your accountability partner can help you with. Seek out what you need or want.

ACTION POINT

OK… You knew I was going to ask this:

Who could you ask to be an accountability partner?

CHAPTER 46

Asking for what you want or need

What do you want or need right now? How hard is that question for you to answer?

"I'd like you to cook dinner tonight, please."

"I need a bit of quiet time to do some reading or writing."

"I want to go to that new coffee shop, not the one we usually go to."

Asking for what we want or need can be quite hard. Perhaps we need to break ourselves in gently. I think, amongst my friendship group, we are getting a bit better at saying no thank you to the things that we don't feel fabulous about.

I love saying if it's a 'hell yes', then it's a yes, but if you're not quite sure about it, then it's a no.

I've grown to love pausing before answering someone's request for my time or energy and I frequently find a loving way to say, "No, thank you."

When practising asking for what I want or need, I find it really useful to add an emotion or feeling to my request:

- "I'm feeling tired, I'd like an early night."
- "I'm feeling fed up, please can you cook dinner?"

- "I'm feeling overwhelmed, I'm popping out by myself for a bit."

A recent client has a family who have decided she needs tough love (whatever the hell kind of oxymoron that is) and she cannot yet bring herself to tell them that she doesn't want or need tough love. She needs really kind, gentle, understanding love. Tough love is making her feel worse. And yet she cannot ask for what she needs at the moment.

Why can't we or don't we ask for what we want? Is it because we fear we will be turned down or otherwise rejected? Is it because we spent our childhoods being told 'I want doesn't get'? Is it because we feel we aren't deserving? Or is it because we are so damn busy trying to meet the needs of everyone else around us? I don't know what your reason is, but I do know mine.

ACTION POINT

Can you start to practise asking for what you want in small ways before you start progressing up to the bigger things?

CHAPTER 47

Revisit and refocus

If you follow sober communities, groups, blogs or podcasts, there's a really common school of thought or piece of advice that's given out to people in early sobriety: get clear on your reasons why you want this (also see Chapter 1).

You want to be sober, alcohol-free, drink less or reduce harm, whatever the right phrase is for you.

Why?

When I first thought about the reasons I had for doing my year-long alcohol-free experiment, I listed my children, my work and my productivity. Of course, I went on to mention my physical health and my emotional health, but they were not my initial thoughts back then. I see things differently now. I only really have one reason why I'm alcohol-free and it's because I want something better for myself. It's so simple now I see it for what it is; I live better this way and I want more of that.

My children, family and friends get the knock-on benefits of a happier, more relaxed, calmer me, but that's a by-product. In the early days of my sobriety, I don't think that I thought I deserved better than I already had. I'd been dealt a series of devastating personal blows a few years earlier and many people would have said my drinking was entirely understandable and justifiable. I didn't have much trust or faith in myself or the world around me at that time – I felt somewhat powerless. I knew that if I carried on drinking the way I was, people would understand. I was numbing and soothing myself and no one would accuse me of being selfish because society allows and encourages us to drink alcohol to get over shock or devastation.

I wanted something better for myself, but I really didn't know if I could have better or if I deserved better. I had had my wildest hopes and dreams granted and then it felt like the rug had been pulled from under me. What if there was more devastation to come? Would I just be laying myself open to further doom?*

So often, our drinking is a reaction to stress, discomfort or worse. It's a tool we pick up without giving it too much thought and it's only when we go to stop that we realise the impact it's having on us.

If we choose to rethink the whole 'why' thing and choose something along the lines of 'because I deserve better', what are the positive thoughts that follow on from that? If I refer to my early list of reasons why I'm not going to drink, we'll find this:

---

* Since that series of 'less than ideal' events in my life there have been more. I'm older and wiser now and recognise that actually sometimes life just has a habit of being 'lifey' and there will always be ebb and flow, dark and light.

I have set myself a challenge and I will succeed with it. I want to be a more patient parent, no more rushing the boys through bedtime because I want to get back downstairs to a drink. I want hangover-free weekends to enjoy my time away from work. I want to maximise my nutritional choices. I want to sleep deeply and wake up feeling great. I want to know I'm giving myself the best chance at not getting high blood pressure, heart disease, liver disease, breast, mouth, throat, oesophagus, liver or colon cancer, dementia or weakening my immune system. I want to know that I'm fun without alcohol.

I look back on that list now and I still feel the same about some of it but, in choosing not to drink, I distil it into just one sentence, and that is:

I deserve better.

Coming to a place of courage to say that out loud has taken time and thought. I've come through the denial stage and learned to trust myself and my judgement more. I really have come so far, and I've got further to go, of course.

ACTION POINT

Where do you stand on the whole 'why I'm choosing to be alcohol-free' question? Is it all about your kids, your wider family, your work? Are you bottom of the list or an afterthought again? Are you often last on your list? Or was that just me? I don't think so.

CHAPTER 48

Be a healthy hedonist

Is there such a thing as a healthy hedonist? Last year, I went on a fabulous retreat in Ibiza… Ah, yes, that beautiful island associated with hedonistic living. Honestly, if I'd been there several years ago, you're damn right, it would have been in pursuit of the utmost pleasure of a different kind. I'd have been leading the charge to the bar, then restaurant, followed by bar, followed by nightclub, I'd have experienced the most enormous hangover and I'd have come home needing at least a week to recover.

Not this time.

The physical and emotional benefits of sobriety are well documented and anyone who doesn't drink will often be keen to tell you about their great sleep, glowing skin, lessened anxiety and non-existent brain fog, but what about the other bits? We are physical, emotional and spiritual beings.

I'm now feeling more and more spiritual connections in my life. Visiting Ibiza was another step in this direction. I spent time in the most amazing villa on top of a mountain with some of my favourite soul sisters, people I've met online and shared life and interests with over the last few years. We ate the most glorious food. We lay in the sun. We did yoga. We meditated. We went for amazing walks to spiritual places. We danced, we laughed and, of course, we cried. We felt connected. Yes to each other, but also to something bigger. This happened not to be advertised as an alcohol-free retreat, but no one talked about drinking as a missing component, I'm delighted to say. I'm well aware that alcohol is low in its vibrational frequency. It is so processed, there's no natural energy in it. Oh, and did I mention the ethanol? Yeah, there's no way that alcohol is a health food. I was so happy to be a healthy hedonist seeking out only good things for my mind, body and soul with other people doing the same.

I love talking about energy and, yes, that is physical, emotional and spiritual too. I'm totally ready to start living in a more connected way now, to slow down more, to listen, to observe, to try to understand. When other people step out, they shine a light on a path for other people to venture onto. I'm not fretting too much about trying to work it all out yet. I know that there's good stuff unfolding for me and for those around me. I don't underestimate the power of sharing my journey. I'm grateful for the people ahead of me who've shared their stories, so I don't feel so alone. We can all step forward together so we can speak about what's important to us and let others find us too. To be hedonistic, healthy or otherwise, is to pursue pleasure. We've all got different pleasures in life. Mine include taking time for myself, reading, walking, sleeping, eating well, being with friends or family and enjoying creative activities. I love little solo holidays or days out, meeting other people when I'm there, but signing up by myself.

ACTION POINT

What kind of healthy hedonist or pursuit of pleasure activities do you want? Want to add to your repertoire? Have a mini adventure searching the internet for your next exciting pursuit!

CHAPTER 49

Telling YOUR story

I've got to start this chapter by telling you I really love my husband. He is loyal, kind, gentle, loving and oh, so funny. I'm not telling you this because he's going to read this book, by the way. Absolutely not. He almost certainly won't!

Here are a couple of things it's useful to know about him. Mr W doesn't like silences in conversations. He's a serial gap filler. Our friends say he suffers from foot-in-mouth disease. If there's an opportunity to put his foot in his mouth, he will. He is the worst keeper of secrets you'll ever meet. If you want a piece of news spread everywhere, share it with Mr W and tell him it's a secret. I guess what I'm trying to tell you is… he's a talker, he's a sharer!

Some time ago, we were out for dinner with a group of friends and there was a momentary lull in conversation. Out of nowhere, he suddenly announced, "Oh, who here didn't know that Sarah stopped drinking a while ago? She's teetotal now!"

I sat there with my mouth open. *What? What? Why would he do that?* There followed a – guess what? – awkward silence. How ironic that the person who doesn't like awkward silences is able to create them so amazingly well.

No one really knew what to say, it was such a random announcement! So, the conversation moved on, in a slightly stilted way, he said nothing further, and I sat there fuming. I waited until the next day to bring it up with him. "I don't like you announcing information about me to a roomful of people. And never use the word teetotal when referring to me, you haven't just walked out of the 1950s," I said. He got a bit narky because he felt that he should be able to say what he liked. I told him that my choices about alcohol were off the table as a discussion point initiated by him, and I thought that was the end of that... until we were away visiting family at Christmas.

We were in Glasgow visiting a large number of aunts, uncles, great aunts, great uncles, cousins, second cousins, first cousins once removed, you get the picture. After a pandemic-dictated break of over two years, we were back! We were hanging out with a bunch of the cousins one day, who are all mostly in their thirties and forties, and there was a lull in conversation. Oh God, you've guessed it. You know what happened next.

"Oh, guess what? Since we saw you last, Sarah has stopped drinking and now she's... she's..." He paused. He panicked. He looked at me. I have no idea to this day what word he was going to say next. He was, sort of, saved by one of the cousins filling in the blank.

"... boring," a cousin finished!

There were a few laughs, a few snorts, no questions and the conversation moved on. I was furious. Again.

I left it until the next day and then I really told him how

I felt. "Do not ever do that to me again, I am not a lull-in-conversation filler. You don't tell other people about the decisions I am making to my lifestyle uninvited."

At this point, I could tell you the things about him that I gave as examples of what I would never talk to people about but I won't do that because that would be me telling you his story and that's not what we're aiming for here. My story about why I decided to stop drinking for a while is mine. My story about how I feel about it is mine. My stories and who I tell them to are personal. I am not a monkey in anyone else's circus. Sure, my decision to stop drinking might have an effect on Mr W, and he's welcome to tell that story, but dangling a piece of information about me and then wanting to orchestrate a conversation or hear other people's opinions... that's not OK. I think I got through to him that time. I cannot guarantee he won't do it again but here's hoping.

I feel most powerful when I have control over my story. When I get to take part in the conversation and confidently contribute. Not when I'm cast as a side character in someone else's narrative.

ACTION POINT

Do other people ever tell your sober story? Do you let them? Are you OK with that?

CHAPTER 50

Are you tired?

It was an average Monday and one of my sons had some homework to do, which he was finding particularly hard. Instead of getting on with it, he kept getting distracted by his phone. To cut a long, tedious and slightly horrific story short, I lost my temper with him and he threw his tablet off the table. Oh, what a joy!

We both fumed at each other, and both felt dreadful afterwards. Meanwhile, my other son was supposed to be in the shower but had actually locked himself in the bathroom and was watching video clips of people playing online games. I asked him to open the door and give me his phone twice. On the third time, I shouted at him and hammered on the door until he opened it and gave me his phone. At this point in proceedings, I had collected two phones, two tablets, a video game controller and my sanity. I was about to go and hide for ten minutes in my bedroom when I realised the TV had been turned on and the online video clips had been sourced on a different screen. I turned the wi-fi off at this stage and then went up to my room, found a large packet of chocolate-covered peanuts that I'd hidden since Mother's Day, sat on my bed and ate the lot.

I'm very conscious of my emotional eating patterns and so I managed to feel both calmed by the chocolate and also horrific at the same time – quite an achievement, I'm sure you'll agree. I then read a chapter of my book to soothe my soul. My husband was out for the evening, so I was freestyling my parenting. Mr W and I are usually a very compatible parenting duo. We can see when each other are reaching points that are bound not to be helpful or useful with the boys and a moment like the one I had just experienced would normally have been seen off because Mr W would probably have found a perfect distraction technique in the heated moment. (Hats off to all solo parents everywhere every damn day.) So, I'm upstairs reading and scoffing chocolate. The boys have no screens.

I did not have a glass of wine to turn to, the glass that might have said, "God, you've survived a less than ideal bit of parenting, well done."

The glass that might have said, "Holy cow, parenting is bloody hard work sometimes."

The glass that might have said, "You deserve this."

The glass that might have said, "Relax, take a load off. You need some me time."

The glass that might have said, "You are knackered, drink me. I'll make you feel better."

You see, the answer to tired/knackered/overwhelmed is never alcohol.

The answer to tired is rest.

But wait, let's get specific here. Let's ask another question. Are you physically tired or are you emotionally tired? Maybe you're both? Well, on this occasion, I was both. I needed to read a book for an emotional break from my thoughts and I needed to sit down by myself as a physical rest.

I had a mini wobble last week because I'd slipped into 'doing' mode. There were errands and tasks, both personal and professional, and it was all becoming a bit much. I caught myself in time – I chose to notice my behaviour, reconsider it and stop doing it. Which is easy to say! The truth is, if you want something to change, you have to choose differently. Every now and again we might need to go back to basics. Basics for me include sleep and rest, movement and nutrition/hydration.

What type of rest do you want or need right now? And what do you need to plan in for later on today? This week, next week, this month? Can you manage to classify it as either physical rest or emotional rest that you need?

I think physical rest is about restoring your body. Sleep, of course, is so important, but there are other tools. Emotional rest is about your inner self restoring who you are on the inside.

Let's list some of them.

Physical rest: might well be deep, restorative sleep, but also naps during the day, and maybe just the act of sitting down and pausing. I used to be terrible for even eating my lunch on the go, standing at the kitchen counter. I was 100% on my feet from early in the morning until late in the evening. No wonder I used to be knackered. What other forms of physical rest can you think of? There's massage, reiki, acupuncture and a squillion other holistic therapies as well. What about yin yoga? Can you move your body slowly and restoratively? How about a form of breathing that you like, just pausing, taking a deep breath? Or practising a particular method of breathing? What about some gentle, slow stretching? Can you take a bath? Can you stop and watch a sunrise or a sunset? If you're feeling unwell or just below par, do you take time off and away from your work? I really hope that you do.

Emotional rest: How can you find peace inside of yourself? Is it music? Is it meditation? Prayer or quiet reflection? Is it in walking or jogging? What about reading a really good fiction book? I love that process of sitting down, opening a book that I'm in the middle of and truly getting lost in it. That is a time for me when I let go of the other thoughts racing around in my head. Can you give yourself a break from technology? Sign out of your social media accounts, perhaps for a day, or maybe a bit longer. What can you do that's creative? Would you like to draw, paint, knit or garden? Something that you can really get lost in. Say no. If you've got enough on your plate already, you don't need to add more things in if you don't have to. Essential oils or flower remedies – have you ever dabbled with those? These are things that I love, I count them as tools in my emotional toolkit.

ACTION POINT

You don't need wine when you're tired, it's a depressant. You do need something else. Think about it, identify it and then take the action. You are so much better than alcohol when you're tired.

CHAPTER 51

Processing your feelings

Have you come across the feelings wheel? (See Action Point). The feelings wheel is a really useful tool for helping to identify and label your feelings, to help you bring awareness to the emotion that you might be experiencing in a particular moment. One of the examples that I give from my early sobriety was that I spent a lot of time feeling angry and I used the word angry because I wasn't quite sure what else it could be that I was feeling. Upon closer examination of my feelings, I found that the feeling I was actually experiencing was one of frustration. So please, look at the feelings wheel, see if it's useful to you. If it is useful, use it, and if it's not, you can put it to one side because there are lots of different tools and modalities that you can try and test and find what suits you best.

Looking at the wheel now, do you have some idea about some of the feelings and emotions you are having at the moment? What about the behaviours that are coming from those feelings that you're having?

I like to consider my feelings from a mind, body and soul point of view.

These are some ideas that are helpful to my mind:

- Writing it down: writing about your feelings and emotions, either in a journal, in a notebook, perhaps just on a scrap of paper (anything that makes that mind-hand connection), allowing those feelings out on to paper is useful. Paper is often a really good starting point for sorting out what is going on inside your head. I love to doodle, scribbling around the side of the things that I'm writing down in any given moment.

- How about something creative: drawing, painting, sewing, knitting. The act of our hands being busy often brings a bit of space and clarity in our mind where we can start to unravel some of the stuff that's going on.

- Talking: I talk a lot about talking! Have therapy, CBT, EMDR, whatever you've tried before that has worked, or try something new. If you've never tried talking before then do! Find a friend who is really good at listening, somebody who can hear you speak about what is on your mind and not make any judgements.

Let's talk about processing feelings in your body next.

Have you ever stopped and thought about where in your body you feel particular emotions? I know, for me, that angry is a feeling I feel in my chest. It's a contracted feeling. My shoulders round, my head comes down. My body feels stiff, the opposite of soft and easy to move. I notice where an uncomfortable feeling is in my body and then I see if I can make some sort of movement or stretch to start to release that feeling.

What about crying or laughing? If you can do those

things spontaneously related to the feeling then fabulous. Or if you need to watch a really sad movie, or perhaps a really happy/funny movie, then go ahead and do that.

And what about your soul?

What are the things that you can do that feel good for your soul to start to sift through your emotions? Meditation, listening to music, breath work – would any of these feel good to you? If they do, then start to use them, and carry on using them if they feel fabulous. And just put them down gently to one side if they don't work for you at the moment.

After trying some of these activities, how do you feel? Do you feel emotionally lighter, mentally clearer? Perhaps you feel more relaxed, or something else entirely. And don't forget that any emotional discomfort you had before might take a little while to process, it might not be a quick fix.

I know that I spent many years escaping, denying, trying to push down, trying to tolerate, trying to control the feelings and emotions that were uncomfortable for me, and coming to a place of being able to tolerate or embrace the feelings took time and conscious effort.

ACTION POINT

Feelings Wheel

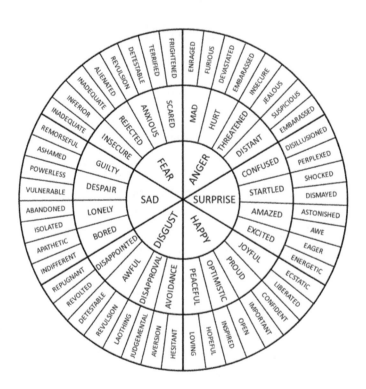

www.drinklesslivebetter.com

CHAPTER 52

Positive visualisations and affirmations

Know what you want from your alcohol-free life, describe your vision in detail (in your mind, written on paper, drawings, poetry) and feel the emotions of your visualisation.

Here is a way you might use a positive visualisation:

- I am going to the pub on Friday night with my girlfriends.
- I will call my best friend the day before to let her know I won't be drinking as I am doing an alcohol-free challenge this month.
- I will plan to get to the pub ten minutes before my friends so I can get my drink and sit down before anyone else arrives.
- I will drink lime and soda/ginger beer/alcohol-free beer/tonic in a fancy gin glass (have your drink in mind before you go so you don't accidentally slip into an old default drink order).
- Play 'the movie' of your night out with the girls in your head in a positive light so you can 'practise' in your mind the success of the evening before you go.

If you like the idea of a visualisation, practise it as often as you can.

Affirmations support a lot of people when they get started on their alcohol-free experiments. Short, positive sentences really help. E.g., "I am enjoying alcohol-free drinks this month." For an affirmation to work, it helps to use the present tense, state it in the positive and keep it brief and specific.

> "I AM. Two of the most powerful words;
> for what you put after them shapes your reality."
> Bevan Lee

ACTION POINT

Do you fancy having a go at writing or saying some affirmations? Get out your notebook/pen and paper and go for it!

CHAPTER 53

No news

Years ago, I was in the kitchen one breakfast time when a news item about a murder came on. One of my boys started to ask me questions about the incident, none of which I could answer. They were questions about detail, which I didn't have, and also questions about bigger life issues, which, at 7am, I was struggling to get my head around. So, I turned the radio off, told the boys that we would chat about it later, and then removed the radio from the kitchen. I've always had a radio in my kitchen and always listened to a talk-based radio station. So, it felt a bit awkward for the first week or so but, over time, we began chatting more as a family in the mornings because we didn't all have half an ear on the news. A short while later, a friend of mine told me she no longer watched the news and there began a whole new way of living for me. I never questioned her decision or asked for more details about the choice she had made. I knew something in me had flipped. I was no longer going to consume the news. Next time I was going to my car, I took a selection of my old CDs and a charger cable to plug my phone in to listen to audiobooks or podcasts when I was driving around. I always used to watch the 10pm headlines but I decided to leave the sofa at 9.59pm and hop straight into bed at that time. I stopped buying my local newspaper and I stopped buying the Sunday paper that I used to buy about twice a month. I've never had any news apps on my phone or news websites saved, so I was already safe from notifications and alerts.

A friend will occasionally say, "Oh, did you hear such and such on the news?" And I reply, "Nope, I don't watch, read or listen to the news anymore." And then we'd start talking about something else. When the pandemic hit, I questioned my decision. Was I being wilfully ignorant? Well, no, actually, I don't think so. I was working in local government at the time and all my work was face-to-face with very vulnerable young people. My line manager was masterful at protecting his staff team and giving us all the information we needed to do our jobs as safely as possible. There was no way the media – local or national – could have helped me out on that one. I was aware of what was going on because, of course, people told me. Sometimes I was willing to listen to a bit of detail, but mostly not. I don't feel like I'm missing out by not keeping up with the news. I'm acutely aware of what I can control in my life, and I know most of what I would see, read or hear on the news doesn't directly affect me. I came to the conclusion that news usually made me feel less good, not better about the world around me. I recognised that I was not taking the time to see a variety of news sources and get differing views. So, what I was getting was incredibly biased, it was debt, disaster or some kind of controversy on repeat. I was not being uplifted in any way, shape, or form.

I realised that my life is going to be short enough. I sometimes don't have enough time for the stuff I really want. So, why was I wasting a precious second on all of this negative stuff? If I need to know something? Of course, I can go and look it up. My own research will be tailored to what I want or need. I don't feel like I'm missing out in any way. I feel like everything in my life is slightly better without consuming the news in the way that I used to. I save some money, I save some worry, I save some anxiety and I save some time. That's good news!

ACTION POINT

Have you given any consideration to your news or media habits? What might you like to be different now?

CHAPTER 54

Four useful thoughts for time spent with people you are finding tricky at the moment

Here are some ideas about the time that we're going to spend with friends, family or loved ones.

First thought: decide upfront what emotions and feelings you want to experience more of during this time. On my list are the following words: calm, peace, love, kindness, rest, quiet and understated. I can't tell you how much I love the idea of an understated time with family, just the right amount of everything, and not too much.

My second useful thought is to identify the activities that make you feel nurtured and identify the activities that make you feel depleted. Add a few more of the nurturing ones and take out, where possible, a couple of the depleting ones. My nurturing activities are reading a good book, watching a film, staring into the fire or the sunset. My depleting activities are too much time spent away from home, too much time with too many other people (or perhaps not quite the right kind of people) and really any time at all in shops.

My third useful thought is about traditions, old and new. Which are the traditions that it's really time to let go of? Have you always seen your family for a Sunday lunch in the pub? Do you always see a particular friend for an end of the month dinner out? Do you always go to the work night out? If you love them, do them and if you don't, take the time to reconsider what could be better.

My fourth useful thought is: don't have complicated conversations when you're already feeling vulnerable or uncomfortable. If there's something big that you need to discuss within your family, is it possible you could leave it until you've got a stretch of sobriety under your belt? If it's not urgent, it doesn't have to be done this month. Just put it gently to one side.

ACTION POINT

What's on your list for emotions or feelings you'd like to feel when you're with those you've made the time to see?

CHAPTER 55

Word of the year
(and word of the day)

I'm not big on long-term goal setting or action planning. I prefer assessing where I am monthly through the year and adjusting my course in small but meaningful ways as I go. I like to use the beginning of the year for a bit of reflection and note-taking on what went really well. I also like to choose a word of the year. Yes, yes, I know, I know – it all sounds very 'out there', only it's not – stick with me and let me explain.

In 2022, the word I chose was simplicity. I had it noted on the front of my diary, on a sticky note on my desk and on my office noticeboard. There were several times that year when I thought about taking on projects or tasks that would have overcomplicated my life and I returned time and again to the thought, *Does adding this mean more or less simplicity in my life?* And that gave me the next move or direction to face. In 2021, my word of the year was growth. Similarly, it helped me to make decisions and plans based upon where I was and where I wanted to be next. In 2020, my word was energy. That was the year I decided to try a 365-day experiment of not drinking and that worked out really well for me! In 2023, my word has been FOCUS. I've been laser-sharp on knowing what I want professionally and personally, and I know a nice anchor word like this will help me. I love the process of choosing a word and then testing it for a week or so before I absolutely settle.

Much more short-term in thinking is my use of a word of the day. I often write my word of the day on my hand in a marker pen – it serves as an ongoing reminder as to what thoughts, feelings or actions I want to embody for that short day in my life. Only good things have come from me having a WOTY and/or WOTD!

ACTION POINT

Have you chosen a word of the year before? Is now a good time to do so? It doesn't matter if you're partway through the year now – there are no rules, just go ahead and choose something you think might serve you well.

What about a word of the day? Is this an idea you could get on board with?

CHAPTER 56

Slightly less than ideal

Things have happened that are 'slightly less than ideal'. If I've said it once, I've said it, well, quite a few times. I've had to recognise what is in my control – my thoughts, my feelings, my actions; and also, what is not in my control – everything else.

Well-meaning and loving friends and family have said, "You must be devastated. What a nightmare. I don't know how you're coping. Get a second opinion," and other various helpful or not so helpful phrases. All said with kindness, I'm sure. I'm letting most of it wash over me. Each time someone says something like, "What a nightmare," I respond with, "Well, it is slightly less than ideal." I know I've caused some people to pause and others to laugh. I know I cannot control how other people react, but I can give them a bit of a hint as to how I am responding to the situation, and I can try to influence their reactions towards me a little bit.

Baxter, our adored family dog, died. It was so, so upsetting to lose him. I'm choosing words like deep sadness, a hollow gap in my chest and hurting heart. Baxter has seen us through some really tricky times. He was our anchor when one of my sons was diagnosed with type one diabetes and our world looked frightening, unpredictable and uncertain. When another family member was diagnosed with multiple sclerosis just three months after that, it was his furry face that soaked up a lot of the tears.

One surprising thing the sadness brought with it was a very physical feeling. I am so used to feeling OK, fine and content, all of which I find reassuringly physically comfortable, I cannot remember feeling such physical emotional discomfort for a long time.

In the same week, I went to the hospital to collect some pathology results. I had a lump removed about three weeks before and had expected to be told all was fine and that there was nothing to worry about. To cut a long story short, everything wasn't fine and there was something to worry about. The surgeon told me the news and then asked me about my lack of reaction to what I'd just heard. I said, "I'm fine. I don't have a strong feeling. I need some more information to make some decisions, and then I'll be OK." I stopped very slightly short of giving him a teenage shrug and 'whatevs' as a response. There was to be more surgery, more waiting, more results and then radiotherapy.

When we came out, Mr W said, "How are you feeling?" And I said, "I am so sad about Baxter. I just don't have much of a feeling about the surgery and radiotherapy. Other than I know I'll be OK."

I thought about how Baxter wouldn't be at home to greet us, to be cuddled to help us with our news. In the afternoon, I told a friend I was OK. And she said, "Oh, you must be numb. You must be in shock." Actually, I'm not numb, and I'm not in shock. I really am OK. I am feeling that message in my body and my mind, and I promise you, I am OK. I am OK because I'm here right now writing this book and you're OK because you're reading it!

I am OK now and I will be in the future. I've been thinking more and more about moment to moment living and this is what moment to moment living looks like for me at this moment.

In the midst of all this, I had invitations to speak at some fabulous well-being festivals, deliver workplace workshops, publish articles and coach more and more clients.

So, some things are less than ideal, but on balance, lots of good and great things are happening. I'll be OK. You'll be OK. We're OK.

PART 4

ALIGNMENT

"To live in alignment with your Spirit is to live your truth and build your life upon it."
Sonia Choquette

CHAPTER 57

Who am I sober?

Now I don't drink, I've had to face some truths. Some of them have been comfortable, some have become comfortable over time and some, well, they are still uncomfortable. Deciding to have a year alcohol-free threw me into a bit of an identity crisis. I was mostly OK about changing my home drinking identity but really struggled with my socialising identity. Shared boozy experiences were a big part of my life and of who I was or who I thought I was.

I've ended up piecing together a bit of a new identity over time. I've reflected not only on who I had been, but also on who I wanted to be in the future. I took time to explore what I enjoyed, and also consciously began to move away from activities I had stopped enjoying. I also looked more closely at my relationships. Who did I want to see more of and who did I need to move away from a bit. Some of the most surprising support came from the least expected places. I discovered that chaos had been a default position for so long that calmness was unfamiliar. To start with, I had to move slowly towards the identity that I wanted. I accept that some friendships have changed, and some have stayed the same. I've also made new friends since becoming sober and a business owner.

Who am I sober? I'm just someone who chooses not to drink alcohol. I want that to be the least interesting thing about me.

Who am I sober? I am an improved version of myself, more relaxed, more peaceful, more patient, kinder and more content. These were not words I would have used to describe myself when I was drinking. Internal chaos reigned.

Who am I sober? Well, probably the most surprising thing for me is to find myself working as a coach. I spent twelve years as a youth worker and a large proportion of my time was spent talking to young people about their substance use without ever considering my own. When I had got sober and completed my coach trainings and certifications, I couldn't believe what I had achieved. None of this seemed possible a short time ago.

I recognise now that a large part of the 'wooohooo, let me lead the charge to the pub/bar/dance floor' part of my personality looked like an extrovert but was indeed an introvert using alcohol as a coping mechanism in situations where I didn't feel comfortable. I'm really happy to lay claim to my more introvert nature now... let me have all the fun – but please can it be in pairs or small groups, please can it be in the morning or afternoon and please can I go home and have a lie down afterwards – thank you!

If you're struggling to visualise/think about who the sober version of you might be then follow good role models to get ideas – read books (like this one in your hand now!), listen to podcasts (*Drink Less; Live Better*, anyone?) and take action. If you're thinking of taking someone's advice, consider if they are currently where you might like to be, have been in a similar place to you now and you have seen them act with care and kindness towards others they are helping.

ACTION POINT

Who are you sober? How do you feel about finding out? Begin your list of your positive sober traits.

CHAPTER 58

Question: do I have to do this sober thing for ever?

Answer: No

Result: The shortest book chapter ever?

Should we leave it there, or is there room for a bit of expansion here? OK, a few thoughts then...

Let's begin by focusing on the right now. Have you been alcohol-free or drinking significantly less for an extended period of time? If not, then I'd kindly suggest you give it a test drive to really feel and enjoy all the benefits of it.

If you've been alcohol-free for more than a year, then what better question can we ask than 'is this forever?'

How about: do I feel better now than when I was drinking?

For me the answer to that is an unequivocal yes. I know for sure that I'm better physically, emotionally and spiritually for not drinking – so, I carry on.

What are the bits you are missing from your drinking life?

Be careful before you answer this – make sure you're not romanticising or looking back with rose-tinted glasses when you remember the good stuff, make sure you acknowledge the bad.

If you can, pinpoint what you feel you're missing and come up with an alternative that will serve you well. I sometimes feel I miss random, rambling conversations that were only born out of a loss of inhibition and vulnerability, but I've found my people who are prepared to have those conversations with me sober!

Find a way to reintroduce the missing bit into your life. Can you swap your night out dancing for a day rave, can you swap dressing up for a night out for dressing up for a day out, can you swap wine tastings for day spas?

So, back to the question: do I have to do this forever? The answer is still no, but do you want to?

When I decided to try my alcohol-free life experiment, I knew I could easily do a month. I had evidence in the form of Dry Januarys, Sober Octobers and was pretty sure I could do three months or even six, but a year felt questionable, outside my comfort zone and definitely a bit challenging.

Did I have to commit to a year? No, but you might want to. The reason it helped me was because it pushed the decision away. Once I'd got started on a year, I didn't question my decision, I just got on with it.

No one makes us choose the goals we set for ourselves. If 'I'm never doing this again' or 'I'm doing this forever' feels good for you then brilliant – I am delighted for you. Say the words out loud and then back them up with action.

"I'm choosing an alcohol-free experiment for a year"

felt like a good statement to me, a thought I was happy to have in my head. It made me feel full of possibility and led me to behave as if I could do it and feel good about it. I didn't feel trapped, and I didn't feel overwhelmed.

If I'd have given myself a thought like 'I'm never drinking again', that would have led to feelings of being trapped or deprived and would possibly have led to me behaving like a toddler in full meltdown – I don't know, as I chose not to put myself in that position.

Nothing we choose in life has to be forever, we can always reroute, reverse or replan. We can change, we can adapt and we can say what we do want and what we don't want.

We can change our minds about who we are.

I used to be the life and soul of the party, leading the charge to the dance floor and last to leave the pub.

I'm retired from all that now – I'm joyfully retired from all that.

I don't have to do it – but I'm choosing to.

ACTION POINT

What are you choosing now?

CHAPTER 59

Your values

Are you crystal clear on what you value most in life? I used to have a set of values that I thought were my core values: family, adventure, freedom and love. But, these were actually things that I THOUGHT I should say to look acceptable to wider society (whatever that is)! I now KNOW for sure what I value most importantly in life and I review those values regularly to check that they are still true and I am living in accordance with them.

ACTION POINT

There are a host of fabulous online tools to help you identify your values and a couple of my favourites are:

https://www.viacharacter.org/

and:

https://www.16personalities.com/

Enjoy learning about yourself and getting closer to your truth!

CHAPTER 60

Unusual choices

Dry December? It doesn't exactly trip off the tongue, does it? We're not about to see one of the big charities pick up that idea as a sponsorship opportunity. That's because it would be way too 'out there', too unusual, too difficult to sell as a concept, too odd, too hard to explain and frankly unrealistic in their eyes.

When I decided to give myself a break from alcohol, I was planning to start on the 1st of January, but as the clock was counting down, I decided I should actually just start then, in December. I was only 'wasting my own time', as my favourite teacher used to say. When I woke up on the 8th of December, I didn't have a crushing hangover. I seem to remember I had drunk very little because my friend's husband and I were doing a ten-mile run that morning. It felt fine to get up, eat breakfast, run and know the last of my drinking had been done, at least for a while. I was glad not to have a big rock bottom moment that resulted in me having to stop. I didn't tell anyone else my plan. I decided I wouldn't drink in December as a warm up to the whole of the following year sober. Surely, if I could do December, then the start of the next year would be easier, and I think

I was probably right. December could be perceived as the most unusual/difficult month to do sober because of all the socialising, but once I had set my mind to it, I was actually OK. I didn't buy myself any Christmas booze, I made plans for how I would tackle my work night out, my friends' big Christmas night out, my mum-friends' dinner and all the rest of the activities that were in my diary. I treated myself with nice alcohol-free drinks and good food through the month. I educated myself by listening to podcasts and reading inspiring books. A Dry December might sound weird to some, but I enjoy a bit of weirdness in my life. I enjoy being an outlier, now more than I ever did when I was drinking.

A Dry December, then; it's unusual but I'm choosing unusual.

ACTION POINT

Are you unusual? Do you have a rebellious streak? How can you use that to your advantage now?

Chapter 61

Journalling your sobriety

I wanted to be someone who journalled. I could see people around me raving about all the joy and the peace that journalling gave them, and I wanted a piece of that action.

Well, I'm here to tell you that I have not yet become a regular journal keeper, I have had times in and out of journalling. It's served me amazingly well at particular points in my sobriety journey and less well at other times.

I have what I call the 'journal graveyard' on a shelf of my bookcase – there are over twenty journals/notebooks there. There are blank diaries, there are beautiful artistic notebooks, there are prompted notebooks, printed ones, beautifully bound ones, homemade ones, A5 size, A4 size and tiny little A6 ones – a complete and utter mixture. Some of them are full completely. Some of them have one or two pages written in.

One of the things I used to really struggle with was the idea of journal perfection and I could not start writing in a journal because I was afraid of either stuffing it up and writing something that I then needed to white out or rub out, or writing something that I then didn't want somebody to go back and look at later on. I got over the fear of making it not look nice enough by starting to use pencils and, later on, using erasable coloured pens. One of the other tricks I use is to print out small pieces of paper and draw nice borders around them. I then use those to write little slogans or quotes on and I stick those in my journals. My journals have a certain element of 'scrapbook charm' about them, which I really love. I'm happy to doodle in my books as well. I write spidergrams, I draw thought bubbles and add little pictures along the sides and in the margins, just because I think it makes my journals look prettier.

I give my brain space to think while my hand is doodling on the page. I had to get really clear about why I wanted to be a successful journaller. Originally, it was because other people were doing it and I wanted the same, but now my reason is because I love having the record to look back on. I was recently looking through my old journals because I was about to deliver a workshop and wanted to remember how I felt when I had just stopped drinking. It was so good to look back and find out what I was thinking, how I was feeling, what my emotions were at that time. I'm so happy to have a record of that now.

The first type of journalling that I really got serious with is called 'morning pages'. The idea of morning pages was put forward by the lovely Julia Cameron and, if you're interested in morning pages, I would suggest you find her online and have a read about what it looks like. In short, it's three pages, a handwritten stream of consciousness that you do first thing in the morning; you write about whatever comes to mind. I wrote my morning pages for about six months and, while I definitely did get some value out of it at the time, longer term, it was not a method of journalling that worked for me.

After I finished my morning pages, I turned to bullet journalling. I really love bullet journalling for the creativity. It allowed me the space to take that grid page, make it into whatever format I wanted and use it as a record, as far as my mind, body and soul is concerned, for the day. I used it as a bit of a trick tick list and I also used it for recording thoughts of, not only what had gone before and how I was feeling in the present moment, but also what my future plans were and what my goals were looking like at that time. That worked OK for a while. I did a solid four months or so of keeping a daily bullet journal. And then I just got out of practice with it.

The journalling method that has worked really well for me all the way through until now is a daily diary. I like to buy an A5 diary that is one page a day and just fill that one page every day. Some days it is a bit of a stream of consciousness, some days it is more drawing than writing. Some days I use journal prompts to write in it, but mostly, it is just a little record of where I am in a given moment. I aim for progress rather than perfection in my journalling practice and, as long as I just keep going with it, I don't have to worry about it looking immaculate or edit my thoughts and feelings.

ACTION POINT

Journalling is an activity that is best started today! You don't need the perfect notebook or the perfect set of ideas to write down. Put your pen to paper now and see what flows.

CHAPTER 62

How can you get comfortable socialising alcohol-free?

Sometimes what you are most afraid of doing is the very thing that will set you free – this was certainly the case for me.

If you'd have asked me years ago how I felt about going out for a night and staying sober, I'd have told you it sounded boring, stressful and antisocial. And that, my friends, is because I was afraid!

I was afraid that I wouldn't have anything to talk about, the conversation would lull, there'd be no raucous laughter and definitely no hilarious stories of the night before to share the following morning.

I was afraid that, if I didn't drink, I'd be asked about why I wasn't drinking and I'd have to explain with a good reason, other people might think I was odd and I'd feel left out because I was the only one not drinking.

I was afraid because, if alcohol bonded us together on a night out, I'd feel as if I was holding everyone else back from their fun. I didn't want to be judged by anyone else and yet... and yet... I was both judging myself and second-guessing what was going on inside everyone else's heads.

I used to be the one who organised the nights out, was first to the bar or dance floor and sometimes last to leave – I felt I had a reputation to either keep up or slowly change. So, I started to suggest alternative activities to nights out; brunches, visits to nice tea shops and lovely long walks where the conversation was fabulous, no one retold the same story three times, we didn't talk over each other and we didn't lose our chain of thought. No one misses the alcohol on these occasions, and I definitely don't miss the hangovers the next day.

I continued to accept any pub dates friends organised. I didn't want to miss out just because I wasn't going to have an alcoholic drink. I made sure I arrived early and ordered a tonic in a big G and T glass so no one questioned what I was drinking. I love being out in the pub with my friends – the atmosphere, the shared experience, the fun – I want all of that please!

I know this won't appeal to everyone who is perhaps in the early days alcohol-free, but I would urge you not to cut yourself off from your really good friends and to ask for their support when you really need it.

Here is a message I shared in a group of some good friends prior to a big socialising weekend when I had been alcohol-free for about six months (and, by the way, these friends were astonished that I'd stuck to my alcohol-free commitment for so long at that point):

"Hi, I'm so looking forward to our weekend together – I love and miss you all! Just so you know,

I'm carrying on with my 'well-being kick' and won't be drinking when we get together. I'll be bringing some amazing ingredients for mocktail making – so no need to feel sorry for me. I'm still happy to play barmaid – I'll pour anything and everything anyone else wants. I'll still talk absolute nonsense, sing out of tune and dance badly. See you on Friday. Ciao. Sarah"

Of course, we had another fabulous weekend together – sending a warning can be a really useful tool for setting you up for successful sober socialising.

So:

1. Accept the feelings if you feel afraid of sober socials to start with.
2. Consider changing your socialising activities.
3. Warn friends if that feels good for you.

You never know, things may turn out much better than you expected, and you'll always be hangover free the next day – that's a win every time!

Don't forget, you're supposed to change. We are not who we were ten years ago or twenty years ago – change is part of being human and some people are more accepting of it than others. Some people will find it confronting because as things change for you, they think it will change things for them and their relationship with you. Be reassured that this is normal!

Showing up as who we are now and giving indications

of who we are becoming might not always be comfortable, but it will be worth it in the long run.

ACTION POINT

Look at your socialising plans (or make one if you don't have one in the diary yet) and look at how you can make it more comfortable for you.

Chapter 63

Fading affect bias

Fading affect bias is the process our brain goes through to forget or fade out unpleasant memories or emotions.

Fading affect bias will make you think *I wasn't that bad*.

Fading affect bias was deeply unhelpful for me in the early days of my alcohol-free life and I'm so glad I kept a diary/notebook at that time, so I had some evidence to look back on and really appreciate how badly I was feeling.

ACTION POINT

Where can you predict fading affect bias might happen for you? What can you do to support your future self now?

Chapter 64

The view from above
(perspective)

Every action you take in the direction of your dreams is reaffirming who you are becoming next – so keep on keeping on in that direction. Master the art of showing up as the new you!

Human behaviour is complex. Often, we perceive our actions and choices through a narrow lens, limiting our understanding and inhibiting personal growth. However, by cultivating a broader perspective, we can embark on a transformative journey of self-discovery and open ourselves to new possibilities. I believe it is important to embrace a wide perspective on our behaviours so we have a chance to move towards profound personal development.

One of the key aspects of adopting a wider perspective is recognising the power of context. Our behaviours are deeply intertwined with the environment, culture and experiences that shape us. By acknowledging these external factors, we can better comprehend the motivations behind our actions and avoid hasty judgements. Understanding the larger context helps us empathise with others and promotes a more compassionate and tolerant outlook.

We all have preconceived notions and biases that colour our perceptions. However, examining our assumptions and challenging them allows us to break free from limiting beliefs and explore alternative viewpoints. By questioning our own perspectives, we open ourselves up to a world of diverse ideas and experiences. This process fosters personal growth, broadens our horizons, and encourages us to become more open-minded individuals.

Looking at our behaviours with a wide perspective involves cultivating empathy towards ourselves and others. Empathy enables us to understand the emotions, intentions and motivations behind our actions. When we approach situations from a place of empathy, we create meaningful connections and develop a deeper understanding of the people around us.

Self-reflection is a powerful tool in developing a wider perspective on our behaviours. It enables us to identify patterns, strengths and areas for improvement. Through self-reflection, we become more self-aware and can align our behaviours with our values and aspirations. It empowers us to make conscious choices and lead a more purposeful life.

Engaging in diverse experiences is an effective way to broaden our perspective on behaviours. By actively seeking diverse experiences, we cultivate a more nuanced and inclusive outlook, enabling personal growth and fostering a greater appreciation for the richness of human existence.

As our perspective widens, we 'zoom out' and look at where we have come from and where we would like to go. We can begin to see the next clear steps we need or want to take and we can move in the right direction.

Accept that some elements about the future will be uncertain – you can only control your own thoughts, feelings and behaviours – see this as a positive!

ACTION POINT

Can you pick up a pen and notebook and draw a path or stepping stones from where you were to where you'd like to be in the future. Can you fill in some action steps in between?

CHAPTER 65

Integration (or letting it all settle)

Once we have chosen some life upgrades that feel more comfortable, more authentic and more aligned, there will likely be a period of time when we need to settle. I often think that the first year of being sober is about learning to be sober and the second year is about learning how to design the rest of your life.

Experiencing a change in your life can be overwhelming and unsettling. It may leave you feeling lost, anxious and uncertain about the future. During such times, it is important to allow yourself the space and time to integrate – which is a fancy way of saying 'let everything settle'.

Give yourself permission to process your emotions. It is normal to experience a range of feelings such as anger, sadness or confusion in times of change. Allow yourself to express these emotions.

Take care of your physical, emotional and spiritual well-being. Engage in activities that bring you contentment. Prioritise getting enough sleep, eating well, moving your body in a way that feels attainable and enjoy some stillness. Less busy is better!

Create a structured routine to provide a sense of stability

in your life. Establishing daily habits can help bring a sense of normalcy and order while you are calming the chaos.

Lean on your support system during this time. Reach out to friends, family or support groups who can provide a listening ear, guidance or encouragement. Sharing your thoughts and feelings with others who understand and care can help ease the burden.

Remember, everyone's journey is unique, and it's important to be gentle with yourself. With time, patience and self-compassion, you will find a new sense of equilibrium and allow everything to settle after experiencing change in your life.

Finding stability takes time. Be patient with yourself.

ACTION POINT

One of my favourite tools to use is a letter writing exercise. I often write a little note to 'past me' and stick it inside a random page in my notebook to look back on and I sometimes email myself to a future date to give myself a little pep talk.

CHAPTER 66

Activating thoughts

Activating thoughts are the internal or external cues that tell us that having a drink would be a perfect idea!

Internal activating thoughts might be emotions or feelings. Examples are: *I am so happy right now, a glass of fizz would make this moment even better,* or *I've had such a bad day at work, a glass of wine would help me de-stress,* or *I'm so tired, a G and T will really perk me up!*

External activators are times of the day, the smell of a glass of wine, a sunny beer garden, the sound of a fizz cork popping.

Be on the lookout for these creeping thoughts – recognise them and don't ever act on them.

Some people talk about 'triggers' and they are probably the same as activating thoughts. I think the word trigger sounds like an action – I preferred not to think about being 'in action' when I was thinking about pouring a drink so this wording of activating thoughts worked better for me.

"I'm tired and a drink would make me feel better" became observed as a thought and was therefore easier to move on from.

ACTION POINT

Which are the thoughts you would like to observe rather than action?

CHAPTER 67

Do I need a hobby now I'm sober?

If you hang out in the 'sober sphere' for long enough, you'll see and hear the conversations around how much more time you get back in your life once you stop drinking. There's no doubt about it. Alcohol is a massive time thief – shopping for it, thinking about drinking it, drinking it and recovering from drinking it. Very little that's productive or creative gets started, worked on or finished once you've opened the bottle and, of course, time is spent nursing hangovers, low-level brain fog and not quite firing on all cylinders.

One pathway towards recovery and wellness is to use some of that time on your physical fitness. Some people start to talk about marathon training, iron mans, Spartan events, obstacle courses, mud runs and other fitness challenges. I can guess what each of these things are, but I have no desire to learn any more about them.

Recognise you're going to have time available and choose your challenge accordingly. If fitness isn't your thing what is? I like to complete a marathon of marmalade making. I spend hours juicing, pithing and really finely slicing oranges and bubbling the marmalade on the hob.

It's one of my absolute favourite start-of-the-year activities. Ten beautifully coloured, rich, sunset orange jars.

We all have different shaped holes to fill in our lives. We each have twenty-four hours in a day but how we fill those hours needs to feel good for us all as individuals.

There's physical fitness to consider but what else? What other activities give you emotional or spiritual contentment?

Do you have hobbies or pastimes? Some of us found new ways to spend time during the pandemic. There was a surge in sales of books, jigsaw puzzles and board games, we took to picking up old creative activities, cake making and decorating, sewing, knitting, crocheting, bread baking, painting, drawing and a squillion other things. Some of my friends picked up old activities and reacquainted themselves with something they loved but had forgotten about.

I felt frustrated. I wanted an actual hobby, and I couldn't find one that I loved. I just couldn't stick with one thing. I did art at A level, and I consider myself to be creative, so why couldn't I just pick up tools and get on with something? I was cross with myself. Then I stopped and thought about it all. I let go of some old stories and beliefs about myself. I allowed in some new thoughts, feelings and emotions. Was I ready to rethink what I wanted?

I started to feel some compassion towards myself, and after a while, I discovered what my hobby is.

Trying new stuff.

I know that's not snappy and easy to understand like 'knitting', but it works for me. I love trying new stuff. Over the last few years, I've made jewellery, made a macramé plant hanger, painted with acrylics, tried a pottery wheel, embroidered, collaged, kintsugied, coloured and more. Turns out, I LOVE trying new stuff.

I don't have to be brilliant at anything, which the perfectionist in me is delighted about. I can play, I have freedom to explore and either love it or put it down and move on. I let go of expecting fabulous outcomes and create for joy and pleasure. I either explore from equipment I have at home or borrow from friends. I buy kits from independent creatives or ask for them as gifts. I go and join classes for one day at adult education centres. I don't care about the cost because I'm not spending my cash on vino any more.

ACTION POINT

Make a note of what hobbies, sports or pastimes you enjoyed as a child/teenager.

What do you feel inspired to try now?

CHAPTER 68

Calm

Be calm. You can, right now, in this moment, choose to be calm. It can be difficult to find moments of calm and serenity. When we're going about our busy lives, our heads may be full of mental to-do lists that we must keep ticking off, the demands that others make of us and the thoughts and feelings we are processing in any given moment.

Let's take a minute now to remind ourselves who we are and what we really value.

Take a deep breath in and out.

Read and say out loud…

I am calm.

I am safe.

I let go of stress.

I choose quiet.

I am peaceful.

I only need to take one step at a time.

I deserve to rest, I can stop.

I am secure.

I choose kindness for myself and for other people.

I breathe out stress and I breathe in peace.

I speak to myself with love.

If I need it, I can ask for help.

It's OK for me to take a break and rest.

I deserve to feel at peace.

I'm not responsible for the things I cannot control.

I invite joy into my life.

I don't need to prove myself to anyone.

I am doing the best I can.

I choose creativity.

It's OK to say no.

I will have a peaceful day.

My thoughts don't rule me.

I'm able to let go of tension.

I can be grounded in this moment.

I am capable.

I let go of intrusive thoughts.

I choose simplicity.

I am loved.

I choose connection with other people.

I deserve self-compassion.

I am calm.

Right now, right here in this moment, I am OK.

ACTION POINT

Read this chapter again!

CHAPTER 69

Can't vs won't

There was something I was stuck with. I listed the reasons why I couldn't start it, which included everything you'd imagine, from time, to energy, to, I don't know, the tilt of the planet or something. Really, it's embarrassing to confess to. Anyway, the real reason I wasn't getting the thing done was a mixture of I didn't want to, I couldn't quite be bothered and there was other stuff. I wanted to do more. I chatted all this through with a lovely colleague, and then felt much better about not doing the thing I didn't want to do in the first place.

When I was first considering going alcohol-free, I had a whole host of reasons as to why I couldn't do it. I was sure I'd be unable to relax, unable to go out with my friends and unable to have any kind of fun ever again. In short, I was going to be miserable.

One day, I decided to switch my language. Instead of saying, 'I can't go alcohol-free', or 'I can't be sober', I started to use the word 'won't'.

Oh, oh, revelation, shocker! When I used the word 'won't' it brought into sharp focus the victim mentality I had been in.

"I can't stop drinking," sounds like 'poor me'.

When I changed to using the word 'won't', it made me realise how much power I had.

"I won't stop drinking," sounds like I was making an active choice to do myself harm.

All this made me realise I was deliberately keeping myself stuck. 'I won't' meant I was choosing on purpose. In the same way I might have said, "Oh, I can't record a podcast, I don't have the time," could have been translated to, "I won't record a podcast because I'm not prioritising it."

When we replace can't with won't, we usually get much closer to the truth and that's a good (if painful) thing. Even if it's a little bit uncomfortable, the word won't puts you in a position of power. You're no longer in victim mode. It's about stopping making excuses, taking responsibility for your behaviour and doing the next right thing for yourself.

ACTION POINT

What is it for you?

Are you saying you 'can't' stop drinking? Do you mean you 'won't' stop?

CHAPTER 70

Are you happy?

Well, it's a really simple question, isn't it? Are you?

Does a simple answer spring to mind?

'Yes, I am happy' or 'No, I'm not happy'.

A friend posted a meme on Facebook the other day. It was a quote attributed to Heath Ledger: "Everyone you meet asks about your career, whether you're married, have kids, etc. As if your life has some kind of grocery list. But no one ever asks if you're happy."

So, in this post, my friend asked the question: are you happy?

He got lots of answers, some predictable, some not so much. My answer was, "I'm happy right now, but I spend a lot of time feeling content, OK, fine and sometimes a bit sad."

I also asked him if he was happy.

It is just one feeling, just one of many, many different feelings that we get to experience. Don't get me wrong, I think it's a lovely feeling and I'd choose it over a whole host of other emotions any day of the week but sometimes it feels like a pretty high bar to reach.

Content, OK and fine are probably the feelings that

I feel most of the time. I consider happy to be a quite elevated feeling. Content happens to be one of my most favourite feelings. I love the cosiness of it, the simplicity, its unsurprising nature. Content feels like there is nothing wrong. No emergency, no immediate danger or threat to life, but a feeling in which I can flow into a task, relax into a rest or look around and know that most things are pretty OK or OK-ish.

Here's another good word: OK. OK isn't given enough kudos, I don't think. OK is such a good way to be. I'm reminded of the old agriculture cultural phrase 'fair to middling, middling to fair' when I describe something as OK. It's average, neither one thing nor the other, it's acceptable, it's passable, it's so-so, all of which I like.

How do you answer the question? How are you? I spent years saying, "I'm good, thanks," because, you know, that's what all the kids were saying, but I've gone back to my roots and the chances are, if you ask me how I am now, I'm much more likely to tell you, "I'm fine, thank you." I downgraded from good to fine a couple of years ago. I'd had a particularly shocking and traumatic series of events in my life and saying good was no longer an answer anyone believed when I said it. Feeling fine rates highly on my feel-o-metre; fine, OK, content, I like them all and they seem so much less pressurised than happy.

I love all the emotions I associate with feeling happy; optimism, excitement, hopefulness and joy. Joy, that's my favourite. I love those total moments of bliss. When you almost feel your heart squeezed for a moment. When you take a deep breath and cannot believe this love-filled moment is real. I accept that those moments are fleeting, they're supposed to be, they are part of the ebb and flow of life.

So yes, I'm happy sometimes, but I'm also delighted to experience all the other emotions that are available to me. I won't label the emotions themselves as good or bad because they are just what they are – indicators, signposts, opportunities to stop, observe and learn from, lean into or adjust. My feelings and emotions affect my behaviours and I absolutely know my behaviours – both towards myself and others – really matter to me and what I value. Are you happy? What feeling are you experiencing? Is that OK?

Also, please know you don't have to try and make other people happy – that is their work, not yours!

ACTION POINT

What needs to be changed in your life to help you experience more of the feelings that you want?

CHAPTER 71

You can't stress yourself to peace

I know this to be true. I've really stressed hard about not having a peaceful life! I love a peaceful life, totally drama free. Who doesn't? Well, actually, me also, but an older version of me. I used to thrive in a zone of slight chaos and overwhelm. Part of my identity was busy-busy-busy and also being anxious about being busy. Not any more, friend, not any more. I love peace. I love calm, and as you may know, if you've been in my world a while, I love contentment. Contentment feels so deeply satisfying to me. My mind feels steady, my body can find stillness, and my soul shines a bit brighter.

How do we move from chaos and overwhelm to a more tranquil way of being? I am afraid we cannot stress, strive, work hard, study deeply or walk over hot coals to get to it. No, it's another way.

For me, it began in about 2018, identifying someone ahead of me on the journey towards less overwhelmed and following closely behind them. I recommend you look for a bit of inspiration online or in real life, find someone being/modelling 'who you want to be' and ask them how they do what they do or how they got to where they are.

Also ask yourself some good questions. I was curious about what was making me feel less than fabulous and some of the answers were feeling tired, feeling like I didn't exercise or eat well enough, not having a passion to pursue and not learning new skills. There was too much of the colour grey, watching or listening to the news, doom-scrolling social media, oh, and alcohol as well, to name just a few.

If there is a list of less than fabulous pointers, there must surely be an opposite. Yes, things that bring me contentment and satisfaction. And those are silence and stillness in my day, reading a fiction book, a bunch of cheery daffodils, a blanket with a hot water bottle in winter and a cool breeze on a warm day. A lovely, scented candle, at least eight hours of sleep, a long, long walk, preferably around twenty kilometres with a lovely tea and cake shop about fifteen kilometres in. Always a yes to the tea and cake. Writing in my notebook, making a rough plan for the day, coming to a place of acceptance that things don't always feel comfortable. There's illness, there's surgery, there's relationships ending, and some things are deeply and horribly uncomfortable. But I found a level of peace in knowing what I can control or influence and what I can't. Finding peace. It's crept up on me gently. I used to chase it hard and be left feeling a bit hollow, but over the last few years, I let go of my desperate need for peace. And you know what? One day I looked up and I had it.

If you cannot find peace within yourself, you will not find it anywhere else.

ACTION POINT

What might you be able to let go of this week? What will help you to allow more peace in your life?

CHAPTER 72

Balance

One of the ways I keep my personal and professional goals aligned is to check once a month how I am feeling about each area of my life. I use a life wheel that looks similar to this one below and rate each area, so I know what I need to concentrate on for the month ahead.

A coaching life wheel is a useful tool used to assess and evaluate different areas of your life in order to identify areas for improvement and to set goals.

Draw or print a life wheel template: Each section represents a specific area of your life that you want to assess and focus on. You can customise the sections based on your specific needs and priorities.

Rate each area: Look at each section of the wheel and rate your level of satisfaction or fulfilment in that particular area on a scale of one to ten, with one being the lowest and ten being the highest. Consider how satisfied you are with your current situation, progress or overall well-being in each area.

Connect the dots: Once you have rated each section, go ahead and connect the dots or draw a line from each rating to create a new perimeter for your wheel. This will form a visual representation of your life balance.

Analyse the results: Take a look at the shape of your wheel. Is it balanced or uneven? Notice which areas have lower ratings and may require more attention. Reflect on why certain areas have lower scores and how they might be having an impact on your overall life satisfaction.

Set some goals or action steps: Based on your analysis, identify specific goals and action steps to improve the areas of your life that scored lower. Think about what you can do to enhance your satisfaction and bring more balance to those areas. Break down your goals into manageable tasks and set deadlines or timelines for each.

Track progress: Regularly revisit your life wheel and update your ratings. As you make progress and take action towards your goals, your ratings in different areas may change.

Use the life wheel as a tool to track your growth and measure your improvement over time.

The coaching life wheel is a visual representation that can help you gain insights into different aspects of your life and guide you towards creating a more balanced and fulfilling life. It's a tool for self-reflection, goal setting and monitoring progress.

ACTION POINT

Life Wheel

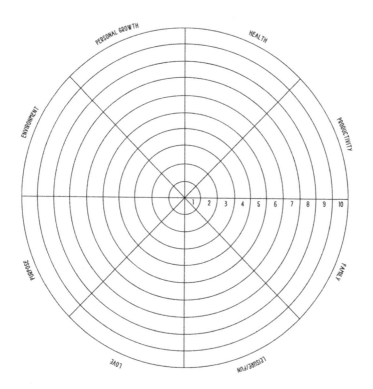

Fun times

Street parties, garden parties, afternoon teas, summer barbecues, festivals and Christmas – we could list so many different gathering types! When a year stretches ahead with the many socialising opportunities, there are loads of types of invitations we receive and perhaps send that we might now like to give a bit more thought to.

We've had a few street parties on my road in the last few years. In the past, I've got involved with organising, but recently I've chosen not to. I swerved the organising completely and, in fact, we went out for the day and didn't attend! What do you do when someone mentions a street party? Are you delighted?

In the run-up to the Queen's platinum jubilee celebrations, I was chatting to clients about their sober strategies. One client said she was going to a party on her mum's street, so she had to drive there and back and therefore can't drink. One client was worried about a party at hers that might have turned very boozy, so she decided on the idea of a morning party with coffee and French toast so there was no need to offer any alcohol. One client chose to go to the cinema to avoid the whole thing. Another drew the blinds and had a home spa day. I love all these ideas. Just because we are invited to things, doesn't mean we have to go, and when we choose to invite other people to our events or gatherings, we don't have to serve alcohol. Here's a fun fact – did you know that garden parties at Buckingham Palace include beautiful plates of sandwiches, cakes and cups of tea or coffee, but no alcohol is served? If that's good enough for the royals' back garden, it's good enough for mine.

When we get a bonus jubilee or bank holiday day, what do you look forward to most? I'd care to bet it isn't a stonking hangover! Is it time away from work? Is it time to spend with friends and family or people in your community? Is it bonus time to spend doing something utterly lovely? Not that friends and family or community aren't lovely. The point is, what do you really want to do? Identify that, do it and don't feel the need to justify it to anyone else.

What about Christmas traditions? They'll be both old and new. Are there any traditions that it's really time to let go of this year? Last December, I got our Christmas tree out and I decorated it but I put the bag back in the loft that had all the garlands and miscellaneous random decorations in it because I just didn't feel like putting them up. I didn't have any judgement about going against any kind of decorating tradition and I don't care if anybody else has got any judgement about it.

A new tradition I've taken on is keeping my Sundays free in December. Last year, I very intentionally left

Sundays activity free in the diary. It meant we could make last minute entertainment decisions as a family. We enjoyed a Sunday where we spent the day with extended family completely unplanned and unstructured, we had another Sunday where we took our boys shopping because it's what they wanted to do. It was lovely. We didn't have anything that we had to say no to and we could just say yes to ourselves.

Try not to have complicated conversations around the holiday season. If there's something big that you need to discuss within your family, is it possible you could leave it until the New Year? If it's not urgent and it doesn't have to be actioned this month, just put it gently to one side.

Please remember that Christmas is often a time away from what you usually do but, while it's your holiday, it is also other people's. In the past, I was guilty of trying to get my family members to indulge in my idea of what Christmas should look like and that might have involved eating Christmas lunch and then playing family games, but not all of my family love playing family games and now I embrace the idea that we're all happily-ish under the same roof together. Somebody might be reading a book in front of the fire, somebody else might be drawing in the den, somebody else might be doing a jigsaw puzzle in the kitchen. We're all doing our own thing. It's not forced fun together, and we're all relaxing and peaceful in the same space. And that is enough. That makes my holiday happy, and it makes everyone else's holiday a bit more relaxed.

ACTION POINT

What social events are coming up and what can you put in place to increase you feelings of contentment?

Chapter 74

Here's the answer you're looking for!

Have you been in the situation where you've told your friends that you're having a bit of a break from alcohol, and they've asked, "How long for?"

"I don't know," is a really good answer.

It means they cannot have an opinion as to whether the time period is too long or too short, they cannot tell you they wouldn't/couldn't do it and they also cannot say that they've got a better idea.

"How will you be able to enjoy nights out sober?"

"I don't know, but I'm going to have fun finding out."

"What will people buy you for your birthday if they can't buy you wine?"

"I don't know, but I guess I'll see when it comes around to it."

"What will you drink on holiday?"

"I don't know, but I'm sure there are always people drinking something who are pregnant, driving or on medication."

"Do you have to do this sober thing?"

"I don't know, I probably don't HAVE to, but I want to."

"What will other people think?"

"I don't know and it's none of my business. They're going to think whatever they're going to think any way."

"Won't you be miserable?"

Oh, for goodness' sake!

I'm not going to say, "I don't know," to that question. No, I won't be miserable, lonely or boring. I'm just going to do a little alcohol-free experiment. This is a choice I'm making from a position of power, not rock bottom.

The sentence, "I don't know," has brought me a lot of head space over the last year or so. I first started using it with my family. I was feeling overwhelmed by the things I needed to do on a day-to-day basis and the emotional energy I had been expending on answering endless questions wasn't helping. So, I started to engage the 'I don't know' strategy. I used the IDK answer as a short sentence. I never elaborated and I always said it with love.

"Mum, where are my football boots?"

"I don't know." See? No follow up of, "Where did you leave them? Are they in the cupboard? Or have you looked by the back door?"

"Mum, what time is Dad home tonight?"

"I don't know."

I did use slight variations.

"Mum, what's for dinner?"

"I'm not sure yet."

"Mum, why isn't my bike tyre inflating properly?"

"I have no idea."

I expected follow up questions: "Mum, can you find

out? Can you google it? Can you ask someone?"

Those questions never came. The boys became more and more clever about finding their own answers.

I also started using it on Mr W.

"What do you think about that political situation?"

"I don't know."

"Why do you think the dog did that?"

"I don't know."

"Do you think it would be better to mow the lawn on Saturday or Sunday this weekend?"

"I don't know."

It's not that I'm avoiding answering all questions. I'm just saving my energy for the interesting and important ones. I still want conversations and interactions, just less of the brain-meltingly ridiculous ones. No one in my family has noticed the 'I don't know' strategy. I'm about a year into it and it just goes to show that I could have spent many years before batting away unimportant questions about football boots, times, food and other stuff.

I'm keeping the strategy for alcohol-free related questions, too. It continues to work exceedingly well for that. 'I don't know' is my gift of a sentence to you today.

ACTION POINT

Use *I don't know* and thank me later!

CHAPTER 75

Think again

Over the course of a day, we have around 60,000 thoughts. When I read this, I thought, *Oh, wow, interesting. So few!* No, of course I didn't. I have no idea how many thoughts we have. I couldn't even have tried to guess. All I know for the answer to how many thoughts we have in a day is… a lot.

The internal thoughts we have are going to be different for everyone. Mine consist of my mental to-do list. My thoughts around my day, my family, my friends, my professional life and my home. My emotions, new ideas, old ideas, things to look forward to, things I'm reflecting on. What am I doing? Who am I being, what do I want next and what am I sharing with others? I talk to myself, I give myself little pep chats and I also tell myself off. I talk down to myself. *I cannot do this. It's too hard. They won't like what I've written. It's not good enough. My voice is too annoying. No one will listen. It's not worth the effort. No one will see the value. There's no point starting if it is not guaranteed to work out.*

Once I start down this spiral, it is quite easy to keep going down. One thought seems to feed the next and the next. I've learned that the sooner I can stop a thought spiral, the less damage it does. As soon as I notice an 'I'm not good enough' pattern, I stop and think to myself, *Oh, hang on. There it is. Let's have a closer look at that.* Noticing and accepting is so powerful in itself. Every day, the most important person we talk to is ourselves. I really believe that who you are becoming is directly influenced by what you are thinking and saying to yourself.

Let's think about drinking for a moment: *I cannot stop drinking now, my friends will think I've got a problem with alcohol. Being alcohol-free will be too hard. Choosing a sober life sounds like it will be miserable. I wasn't that bad. I could just carry on and only drink at weekends. Perhaps there's no point in starting with this. I'll probably fail.*

Can you choose new thoughts and emotionally connect to them?

Let's try this on for size instead: *I'm choosing new ways of relaxing and socialising. My choice not to drink is a powerful one. I am in control of my actions. I will make progress. I'm on my alcohol-free journey. My success is in my hands. I am taking inspired action.*

Remember that if you do the same as you've always done, you'll always get the same results that you've always got.

ACTION POINT

If now is the moment to think again, do it, rethink it!

CHAPTER 76

Sober socials

Since I chose to be alcohol-free, I've learned a thing or two about how I best like to spend my time and it hasn't really turned out how I would have guessed. I used to be lovingly known as the 'social secretary' within my friendship group and I used to relish that role. Who's up for a Christmas party? Right? Leave it to me. Date, time, venue, menu, drinks sorted. Trip to a Christmas market with mulled wine: invite issued. New Year's Eve games, food, drinks, done. Random nights out for dinner, drinks, theatre trips, comedy events, birthdays. I'm your organised friend, you say yes and we're off!

It's not like that now. A walk? Yes. A coffee date? Yes. Occasional brunch or lunch? Yes.

Dinner? Rarely. What happened? Well, I found out a bit more about myself and, while it took me a while, I grew to like me. I prefer mornings and walking. I prefer hot drinks and chats. I prefer evenings in. I love seeing my friends one-to-one or in small groups. After years and years being happy in my oldest friendship circles, I'm actually enjoying making lots of new friends at the moment. My advice to you is to carry on socialising as you always did. But when you go out, ask yourself several times, "Am I loving this? Is this bringing me joy? Am I having fun? Is this what I want to be doing with my time?" If it is, great, if not, offer your friends other suggestions. The activities that don't centre around drinking, they might just want a break too. Something that has surprised me is just how much I love time alone. Recently, I was gifted a night in a hotel about an hour from home. I loved the solitude, the freedom to do what I wanted, eat when I wanted and to generally please myself. "Won't you feel lonely if you go by yourself?" someone asked me. Absolutely not! So, switch it up, friend. Check in and see how your social time is spent.

ACTION POINT

Make some new suggestions to your friends. Try new things and then see how you feel about it all.

Chapter 77

When you are having one of those days...

Today is just one day, it's just one day; yesterday was just one day as well.

One day, with twenty-four hours, approximately eight of those sleeping.

One day, perhaps with three meals.

One day, perhaps with some work.

One day, perhaps with some daily tasks.

One day, perhaps with some time alone, some time with other people.

One day to choose gentle, choose soft.

Choose to be kind to yourself.

What are the choices you would like to make on this one day?

I choose to be alcohol-free. I choose to do some of the work I love. I choose some creativity. I choose time alone to read. I choose time to connect with other like-minded people.

Whether we are alone or surrounded by others, it's easy to get fooled into thinking we need alcohol to help us shift our emotions, but have you stopped to closely examine your emotions?

Are you lonely or isolated? Are you bored? Are you frustrated? Overwhelmed, disappointed or worried?

What are the ways you can bring relief into your life? Can you call a friend or indeed call someone else who you know might also feel isolated? Can you choose a boredom relieving activity? Can you put on some high vibe music, dance, walk, exercise, take a bath, shut yourself in a bedroom for ten minutes?

Whatever emotion you are feeling, check in and see what fits as a feel slightly better activity.

Can you do that for just one day, just today?

Go with it. Minutes turn into hours, the clock will tick, the light will fade. You will go to sleep, and you will wake up again on the other side.

I wish you peace. I wish you hope. I send you love today.

It's OK. You are OK.

ACTION POINT

Some days we MUST choose kind, gentle softness. We can choose love and compassion for ourselves, not just for everyone around us.

CHAPTER 78

Moments of bliss

I think we've put a high expectation on ourselves to be happy and perhaps a high expectation on other people around us to be happy, too. How often have you heard these words: "I just want my kids to be happy." Saying the word 'just' in that sentence makes it sound as if it's a simple thing to want. And the word happy? Well, sometimes that's a big ask, too. It's a big ask for people around us and it can be an enormous ask for ourselves. I'm delighted that happiness is something that I experience in really short bursts. It could be when I'm sitting at the table with friends and family, in that moment where somebody shares a joke and we all laugh, or it could be a shared connection with a friend on a dog walk. All sorts of different things make me feel happy, but I recognise that happiness is quite a short-lived feeling. Most of the time, I'm not living my life feeling happy and, you know what? I'm fine with that. I think that knowing my favourite feeling is contentment has brought me a lot of peace. It's taken me a while to come round to figuring this out. For a while, I saw contentment as being too close to boredom or fed up but, in fact, it isn't that at all for me. Boredom and feeling a bit fed up are actually getting more and more comfortable for me the further along I go in my sobriety.

At the top of my happiness scale, I think of bliss, and I tend to experience bliss in fleeting moments. I've got two different moments of bliss I'd like to share with you. The first one struck me completely out of the blue. It was towards the end of summer; I'd say it was probably late August time, maybe even early September. My boys were playing football with their team, and I was sitting on the side of the field. I can't remember whether the score was going our way or not. I was sitting on the grass, Baxter my dog curled up around my leg. I had a coffee in a takeaway mug I had brought from home, and I was wearing a really colourful pair of leggings. The sky was that gorgeous, gorgeous late summer bright blue with not a cloud in sight. The temperature was warmish. I remember I was wearing a T-shirt, a sweater and a scarf, so it wasn't hot. I remember turning my face towards the sun and suddenly feeling this enormous whoosh. This feeling washed completely up and over me and it stayed for a while. I had my eyes open and then I closed them, took a really deep breath in and let a long breath out. I opened my eyes again and I looked around at this perfect moment. The feeling probably lasted for about thirty seconds and I enjoyed it while I was in it, but I knew it was going to slip away again. However, in that moment, it was pure lightness and pleasure. A few seconds after that moment, I thought, *I'm always going to remember this moment*. I took a photo of Baxter, of the football field, of my leggings. It was a moment that I think of now as shorthand when I think of what bliss feels like.

I had another experience of a moment of bliss more recently. I spent a night in a hotel for a lovely break and the next morning, after I'd had breakfast, I walked into the lounge. I had the book I was reading in my hand and there was an armchair facing a window in a sunbeam. I made a beeline for this armchair, sat down in it and put my book on the floor. I just closed my eyes and I felt that sunshine beating on my eyelids. For a moment, I stared really hard at the insides of my eyelids, and I looked at all of the different colours and then I slowed my breathing down. I was just there in that moment, by myself, experiencing another amazing moment. I took a photo of that chair to remember that moment, too.

There are two of my moments of bliss, both experienced recently, sunshine and colour a recurring feature. In both moments, the sounds around me were happy noises of children and birdsong. In those moments, I felt 100% everything I was supposed to feel, and it was lovely. Be on the lookout for your moments of bliss. See if you can catch them. They might be fleeting but hold on to them, so that you can remember them and reflect on them.

ACTION POINT

Can you remember a moment of bliss in your life? Are you able to 'go back there' and reflect on it/ relive it?

CHAPTER 79

Simple acts of self-love

What can we do for ourselves to bring a little bit more love and care into our lives?

1. My number one tip for you all is: turn off the news (more on this in Chapter 53 No News). I turned off the news a few years ago. I was listening to so much negativity in the morning. My kids were getting ready for school in the kitchen and asking me questions about the items on the news that I couldn't really answer. Every story seemed to be negative; it was not filling any of our hearts with positivity and joy in the morning. The radio in the kitchen was the first thing to go, then the ten o'clock headlines and one day I just stopped listening, watching or reading any news at all. I don't have anything on my social media feeds as far as news is concerned and the only things that I get sent are things by friends or family that they think might be of particular relevance or interest to me. My mum occasionally cuts things out from the physical newspaper and sends them to me. I love that this is a truly edited news feed.

2. Take five minutes to get in the shower. I know at times

in my life when I was feeling really rubbish, the most difficult thing of a morning was getting into the shower.

3. Read a chapter of your favourite book. Now, I love self-development and learning as much as the next person, but I can't tell you what joy I get from reading a really good novel. I go to the library on a regular basis, and I use the app to order the books that I want, which means that they'll be on the shelf waiting for me when I get down there. I love the act of borrowing a book and then taking it back. I don't need to own physical copies of these books unless it's something I particularly love and want to own.

4. A cup of tea. I am the number one fan of sitting in that chair with that freshly brewed cup and just staring at the steam over the rim of the mug, out of the window and really enjoying that drinking experience.

5. Gentle movement of your body in a way that feels right for you, just now. If running isn't your thing, that is fine, move slowly, stretch. Do whatever it takes to really feel into your physical body. I've stopped running now, I'd consider myself to be much more of a walker and I'm all the happier for it.

6. Eat and drink as best as you can possibly manage in any given moment. Don't buy that food that you know you really don't want to eat. I know it's easy to say but try not to do it.

7. Stop the comparison. While it's OK to look at other people who are a few steps ahead of you and desire a bit of what they've got, you do not need to compare

yourself to them. This will only decrease your self-love. You are doing you and they are doing them.

8. Focus very closely on your self-talk. Be as loving and compassionate as you possibly can be to yourself. Speak to yourself how you would a very dear friend.

9. Do find comfort in time spent alone if that feels good for you.

10. Be patient and kind to yourself. Congratulate yourself on all the accomplishments, even the really teeny, tiny ones.

Lastly, do more of the things that you love and, where you possibly can, do less of the things that you don't.

Closing thoughts

Drink Less; Live Better… my wish for you is that by choosing to re-evaluate your relationship with alcohol you will automatically live a better version of your life. My life is so much more manageable without alcohol. I have calmed some of the chaos and feel better for it. I am still a 'work in progress' as we all are. Choose what you want; peace, calm, joy, fun, adventure, enlightenment or whatever feels good to you and move towards it.

Living a fulfilled life is a pursuit shared by many, remember, it's useful to embrace a holistic approach that incorporates awareness, acceptance, action and alignment along the way. These four interconnected tools serve as a roadmap to navigate life's challenges and cultivate a genuine sense of fulfilment. We can apply these ideas to drinking less, living alcohol-free, changing jobs, evaluating relationships and many other areas of our lives.

AWARENESS

The first step towards contentment is cultivating awareness. It involves developing an understanding of oneself, others and the world around us. By being present in the moment and observing our thoughts, feelings and behaviours, we gain clarity and insight. Self-awareness helps us recognise our strengths, weaknesses, passions and values. It allows us to identify patterns and habits that may hinder us. Additionally, awareness extends beyond ourselves, enabling us to empathise with others and appreciate the interconnectedness of all beings. With awareness, we can let go of judgement and embrace compassion, fostering harmonious relationships and deepening our connection to the world.

ACCEPTANCE

Acceptance involves embracing ourselves and others unconditionally, acknowledging that imperfections are an integral part of the human experience. When we practise self-acceptance, we release the burden of self-criticism and comparison, allowing us to nurture a more positive self-image. Accepting others as they are, without trying to change or control them, fosters deeper connections and promotes more harmonious relationships. Acceptance also extends to circumstances and events in life. By accepting the ups and downs, we let go of resistance and find a level of peace in the present moment. Embracing acceptance empowers us to overcome obstacles, grow from challenges and experience the beauty of life's imperfections.

ACTION

Taking action involves setting goals, making choices and actively pursuing our dreams and aspirations. Action transforms awareness and acceptance into tangible outcomes. It requires courage, determination, and perseverance. By taking proactive steps towards our desires, we create a sense of purpose and fulfilment. Moreover, action allows us to learn and grow, enabling us to expand our horizons and discover new possibilities. It is through action that we turn our dreams into reality and experience the satisfaction of achievement. Every small step we take, no matter how seemingly insignificant, propels us forward on our journey towards a joyful life.

ALIGNMENT

Alignment refers to living in harmony with our true selves and our values. When we are looking to achieve alignment in our lives, we must regularly evaluate and reassess our choices and priorities. Aligning our actions with our values ensures that we live authentically and with integrity. Furthermore, nurturing positive and supportive relationships that align with our values contributes to our overall well-being. When we align our lives with what truly matters to us, we experience a sense of purpose and flow, bringing peace to every aspect of our existence.

Awareness, acceptance, action, and alignment serve as powerful tools for navigating life. By cultivating awareness, practising acceptance, taking inspired action, and aligning our lives with our values, we can unlock the doors to genuine contentment and live a life we are deserving of.

PS… I believe in you.

Sarah Williamson

www.drinklesslivebetter.com
– download the five-day drink less programme

Drink Less; Live Better Podcast
– listen for a weekly dose of kindness, insight and wisdom

Printed in Great Britain
by Amazon